This publication is intended to provide educational information for the reader on the covered subjects. It is not intended to take the place of personalized medical counseling, diagnosis, and treatment from a trained healthcare professional.

ISBN 978-1-998740-13-0 (Paperback)
ISBN 978-1-998740-14-7 (eBook)

Printed and bound in USA
Published by Loons Press

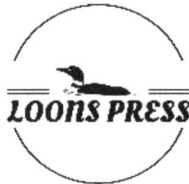

I0106270

LOONS PRESS

Table Of Contents

How To Manage Liver Cirrhosis

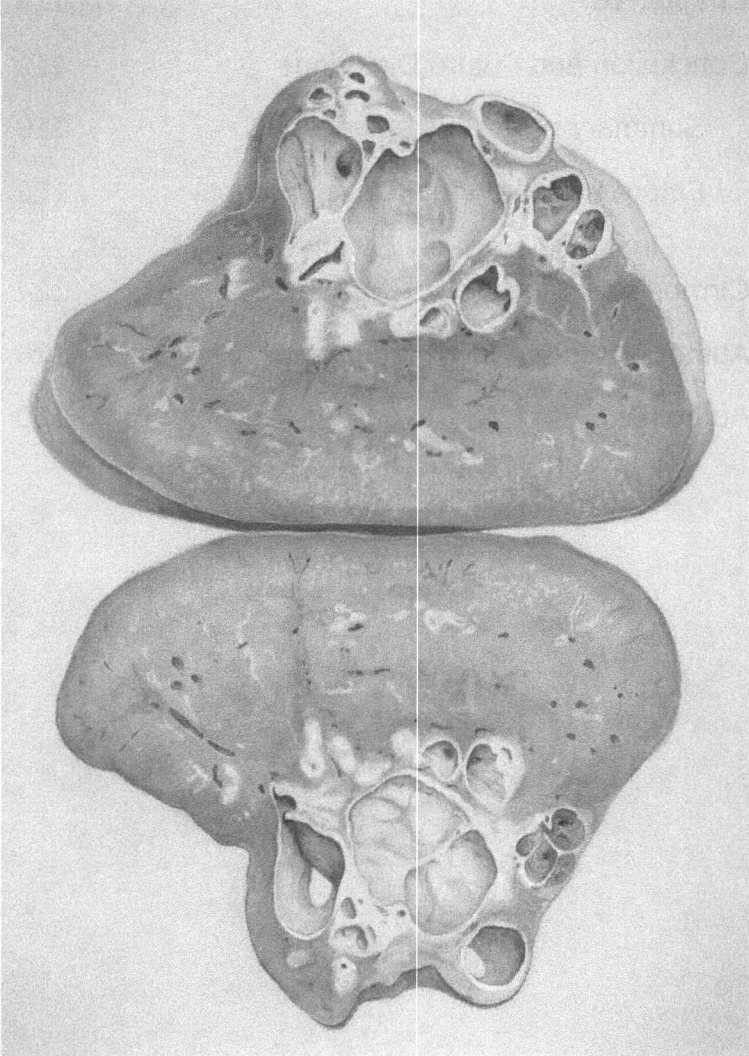

Chapter 1

Understanding Liver Cirrhosis

What is Liver Cirrhosis?

Liver cirrhosis is a progressive liver disease characterized by the gradual replacement of healthy liver tissue with scar tissue, resulting in impaired liver function. This condition often develops over many years due to various underlying factors, including chronic alcohol abuse, viral hepatitis, and non-alcoholic fatty liver disease.

As the liver becomes increasingly scarred, its ability to perform essential functions, such as detoxifying harmful substances, producing vital proteins, and aiding in digestion, diminishes significantly. Understanding liver cirrhosis is critical for those concerned about managing this serious health issue.

The liver is an essential organ in the human body, playing a crucial role in metabolism, detoxification, and the synthesis of various proteins. When cirrhosis occurs, the liver's architecture is disrupted, leading to portal hypertension, which is an increase in blood pressure within the liver's portal vein. This can result in severe complications, including varices (enlarged veins), ascites (fluid accumulation in the abdomen), and even liver failure. The progression of cirrhosis can vary among individuals, and some may remain asymptomatic for years, while others may experience rapid deterioration.

Cirrhosis is often classified into two main types: compensated and decompensated. Compensated cirrhosis means that the liver is still able to perform most of its functions, and patients may not show any symptoms. However, as the disease progresses to decompensated cirrhosis, symptoms such as jaundice, fatigue, swelling in the legs and abdomen, and confusion may arise. Identifying the stage of cirrhosis is crucial as it influences treatment options and management strategies. Regular monitoring and medical evaluations can help detect changes in liver function and allow for timely interventions.

Management of liver cirrhosis involves a comprehensive approach that focuses on addressing the underlying causes, preventing complications, and improving the quality of life for patients. Lifestyle modifications, such as abstaining from alcohol, maintaining a healthy diet, and engaging in regular physical activity, are essential components of care. Additionally, medications may be prescribed to manage symptoms and complications, such as diuretics for fluid retention or beta-blockers to reduce portal hypertension. In advanced cases, liver transplantation may be considered as a life-saving option.

Early diagnosis and proactive management of liver cirrhosis can significantly impact patient outcomes. Education and support for patients and their families play a vital role in navigating the complexities of this disease. Resources, including support groups and educational materials, can empower individuals to take an active role in their care. By understanding what liver cirrhosis is, its implications, and the strategies for managing it, patients can work towards maintaining their health and enhancing their overall well-being.

Causes of Liver Cirrhosis

Liver cirrhosis is a progressive condition characterized by the replacement of healthy liver tissue with scar tissue, impairing liver function. Understanding the causes of this condition is crucial for managing and preventing its progression. The primary causes of liver cirrhosis can be broadly categorized into alcoholic and non-alcoholic factors. Alcohol-related liver disease is one of the most common causes, where excessive alcohol consumption leads to liver damage over time. Chronic alcohol abuse disrupts the liver's ability to detoxify the blood, leading to inflammation, fatty liver, and eventually cirrhosis.

Non-alcoholic fatty liver disease (NAFLD) is another significant contributor to cirrhosis. This condition is often associated with obesity, diabetes, and metabolic syndrome. In NAFLD, fat accumulates in liver cells without inflammation, but it can progress to non-alcoholic steatohepatitis (NASH), causing liver inflammation and damage.

Individuals with insulin resistance are particularly at risk, as the excess fat in the liver can trigger a cascade of inflammatory responses, ultimately leading to cirrhosis if not managed effectively.

Chronic viral hepatitis, particularly hepatitis B and C, is also a leading cause of liver cirrhosis worldwide. These viral infections can cause ongoing liver inflammation and damage that may lead to cirrhosis over several decades. The progression from chronic hepatitis to cirrhosis can be influenced by various factors, including the individual's immune response and the presence of coexisting liver conditions. Vaccination and antiviral treatments can significantly reduce the risk of cirrhosis in those infected with hepatitis viruses.

Autoimmune liver diseases, such as autoimmune hepatitis and primary biliary cholangitis, are additional causes of cirrhosis. In autoimmune hepatitis, the body's immune system mistakenly attacks liver cells, leading to inflammation and fibrosis. Primary biliary cholangitis involves the gradual destruction of the bile ducts, which can also contribute to liver damage.

Both conditions require early diagnosis and appropriate immunosuppressive therapy to manage symptoms and prevent progression to cirrhosis.

Lastly, certain inherited metabolic disorders, such as Wilson's disease and hemochromatosis, can lead to liver cirrhosis. Wilson's disease results in copper accumulation in the liver, while hemochromatosis involves excessive iron deposits. Both conditions can cause significant liver damage if not recognized and treated promptly. Understanding these diverse causes is essential for those concerned about managing liver cirrhosis, as addressing the underlying factors is key to improving liver health and preventing further complications.

Symptoms of Liver Cirrhosis

Liver cirrhosis is a progressive condition characterized by the replacement of healthy liver tissue with scar tissue, leading to a decline in liver function. Symptoms of liver cirrhosis can vary significantly among individuals and may be subtle in the early stages, making early diagnosis challenging.

Patients and caregivers should be aware of the various symptoms to seek timely medical intervention and manage the condition effectively.

One of the most common early symptoms of cirrhosis is fatigue. Individuals may experience a persistent sense of tiredness that is not alleviated by rest. This fatigue can significantly impact daily activities, leading to decreased productivity and quality of life. Alongside fatigue, many patients report a loss of appetite, which can result in unintended weight loss. This change in appetite can stem from the body's altered metabolism and the liver's reduced ability to process nutrients, emphasizing the importance of monitoring dietary intake.

As cirrhosis progresses, more pronounced symptoms may emerge, including jaundice. This condition is marked by a yellowing of the skin and eyes due to the accumulation of bilirubin, a substance produced during the breakdown of red blood cells. Jaundice can be accompanied by dark urine and pale stools, indicating impaired liver function.

The appearance of these symptoms warrants immediate medical evaluation, as they signify significant liver dysfunction and the need for potential adjustments in management strategies.

Additional symptoms often seen in individuals with cirrhosis include swelling in the legs and abdomen, known as edema and ascites, respectively. This occurs due to fluid retention, a consequence of the liver's inability to produce proteins that help maintain fluid balance in the body. As the condition progresses, patients may also experience easy bruising or bleeding, a result of decreased production of clotting factors.

Recognizing these signs is crucial, as they may indicate worsening liver health and the need for prompt treatment to alleviate discomfort and prevent complications.

Finally, cognitive changes may arise in individuals with cirrhosis, known as hepatic encephalopathy. Symptoms can range from mild confusion and forgetfulness to severe disturbances in consciousness.

This condition occurs when the liver cannot adequately remove toxins from the bloodstream, leading to their accumulation and subsequent effects on brain function. Monitoring for these cognitive changes is essential, as they may necessitate alterations in treatment and lifestyle to improve overall liver health and quality of life. Understanding these symptoms enables better management of liver cirrhosis and highlights the importance of regular medical follow-ups for those affected.

Stages of Liver Cirrhosis

Liver cirrhosis progresses through distinct stages, each characterized by specific symptoms and underlying changes in liver function. Understanding these stages is critical for effective management and intervention. The initial stage, often referred to as compensated cirrhosis, may not present noticeable symptoms. The liver, despite being damaged, can still perform its essential functions. Patients may experience fatigue, occasional discomfort in the upper abdomen, and slight changes in appetite. During this stage, routine monitoring and lifestyle modifications can significantly slow progression.

As cirrhosis advances to the decompensated stage, more severe symptoms begin to manifest. This stage is marked by the liver's inability to compensate for its damage, leading to complications such as jaundice, ascites, and hepatic encephalopathy. Jaundice, characterized by yellowing of the skin and eyes, occurs due to the accumulation of bilirubin. Ascites, the buildup of fluid in the abdominal cavity, can cause discomfort and impact mobility. Hepatic encephalopathy affects brain function, leading to confusion and altered consciousness. At this point, medical intervention becomes crucial to manage symptoms and prevent further deterioration.

The transition from compensated to decompensated cirrhosis can vary significantly among individuals, influenced by factors such as the underlying cause of liver disease, comorbidities, and adherence to treatment protocols. Regular follow-up with healthcare providers is essential to monitor liver function and detect any signs of progression early. Patients should be educated about the importance of attending routine appointments, undergoing necessary tests, and maintaining open communication with their healthcare team to tailor management strategies effectively.

In advanced stages of cirrhosis, known as end-stage liver disease, the liver's functionality diminishes drastically, leading to life-threatening complications. Patients in this stage may require more intensive medical interventions, including hospitalization or consideration for liver transplantation. Management focuses on alleviating symptoms, preventing complications, and improving the quality of life. Palliative care becomes a significant aspect of treatment, emphasizing comfort and support for both patients and their families.

Ultimately, recognizing the stages of liver cirrhosis is vital for effective management. Early detection and proactive management strategies can significantly impact the progression of the disease. Patients and caregivers should be well-informed about each stage's implications and remain vigilant for any changes in symptoms. By understanding the stages of cirrhosis, individuals can better navigate their care journey and advocate for the necessary support and interventions to enhance their health outcomes.

How To Manage Liver Cirrhosis

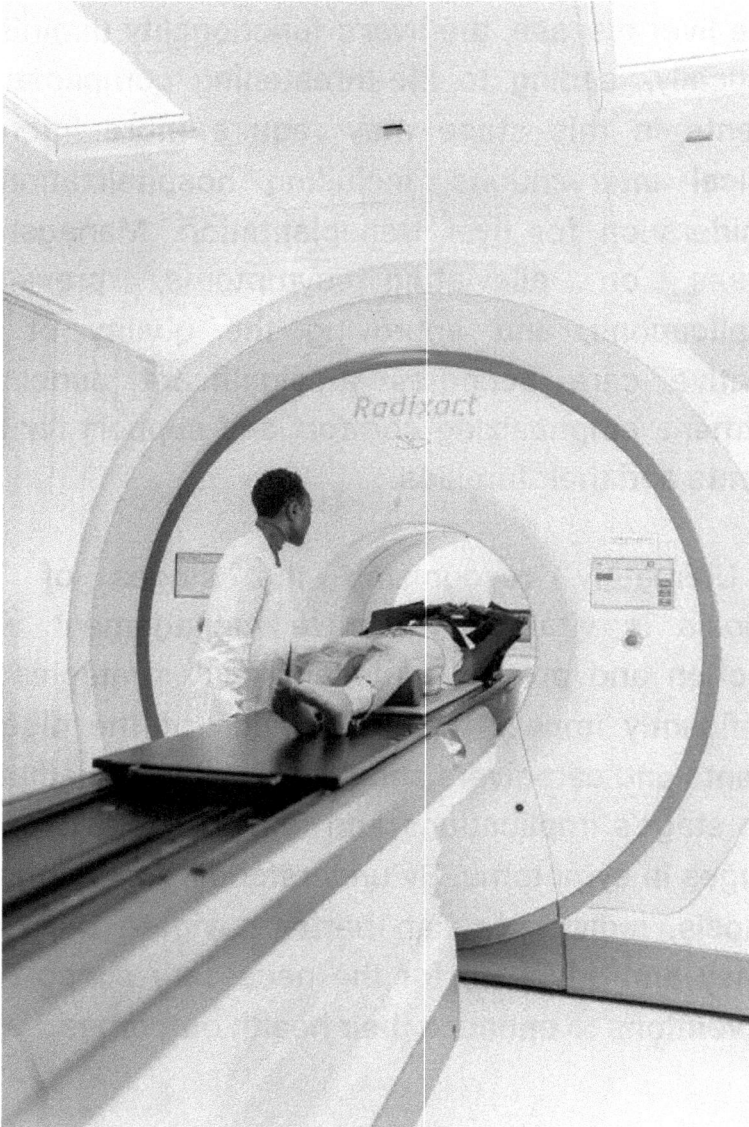

A Comprehensive Guide

Chapter 2

Diagnosis of Liver Cirrhosis

Medical History and Physical Examination

Medical history and physical examination are critical components in the assessment and management of liver cirrhosis. Gathering a comprehensive medical history allows healthcare providers to identify potential causes of liver disease, assess the severity of the condition, and tailor management strategies accordingly. Patients should be prepared to discuss their symptoms, such as fatigue, jaundice, abdominal swelling, and any changes in appetite or weight.

Additionally, it is essential to provide information on past medical conditions, medication use, alcohol consumption, and any family history of liver disease, as these factors can significantly influence the management of cirrhosis.

During the physical examination, healthcare providers will conduct a thorough assessment to look for signs that indicate liver dysfunction. This may include inspecting the skin for jaundice, checking for spider angiomas, and assessing abdominal distension. The examination may also involve palpating the abdomen to evaluate the liver's size and texture, as well as checking for signs of ascites or fluid accumulation. These findings not only help in diagnosing cirrhosis but also provide insight into its complications, which can be pivotal in determining the urgency and type of intervention needed.

Laboratory tests and imaging studies often complement the medical history and physical examination. Blood tests can reveal elevated liver enzymes, bilirubin levels, and decreased albumin, all of which help to assess liver function and injury. Imaging studies, such as ultrasound, CT scans, or MRIs, provide a visual representation of the liver's structure and can identify complications like portal hypertension, liver nodules, or changes consistent with cirrhosis. Together, these diagnostic tools enable healthcare providers to establish a baseline and monitor disease progression over time.

Effective management of liver cirrhosis also requires ongoing evaluation and adjustment of care plans based on the patient's evolving condition. Regular follow-up appointments are essential to monitor liver function, manage symptoms, and screen for complications such as liver cancer or variceal bleeding. Patients should engage actively in their care by reporting any new symptoms or concerns promptly. This collaborative approach between patients and healthcare providers fosters a more personalized management plan and improves overall outcomes.

Finally, understanding the relationship between medical history, physical examination, and ongoing management plays a vital role in living with liver cirrhosis. Patients who are informed about their condition and proactive in their care are better equipped to navigate the complexities of this disease. By recognizing the significance of thorough assessments and maintaining open communication with healthcare providers, individuals can take an active role in managing their liver health and improving their quality of life.

Laboratory Tests

Laboratory tests play a crucial role in the diagnosis and management of liver cirrhosis. These tests provide essential information about liver function, the extent of liver damage, and the presence of underlying conditions that may contribute to cirrhosis. A comprehensive understanding of laboratory tests is vital for individuals concerned about managing liver cirrhosis, as these tests can help guide treatment decisions and monitor disease progression.

One of the primary tests used in assessing liver function is the liver function test (LFT). This panel of blood tests measures the levels of liver enzymes, bilirubin, and proteins produced by the liver. Elevated levels of enzymes such as alanine aminotransferase (ALT) and aspartate aminotransferase (AST) may indicate liver inflammation or damage. Bilirubin levels can indicate the liver's ability to process waste products, while low levels of albumin, a protein made by the liver, can signal impaired liver function. Regular monitoring of these markers is essential for tracking the progression of cirrhosis and evaluating treatment effectiveness.

Additionally, tests that assess the coagulation status of the blood are important in managing liver cirrhosis. The liver is responsible for producing several proteins necessary for blood clotting; therefore, liver dysfunction can lead to coagulopathy. The prothrombin time (PT) and international normalized ratio (INR) are commonly used tests to evaluate the coagulation ability of an individual. Prolonged PT or elevated INR may indicate a higher risk of bleeding complications, which is a significant concern for patients with cirrhosis. Understanding these values helps healthcare providers assess the need for interventions to manage bleeding risks.

Another important set of tests includes those that evaluate for viral hepatitis, which is a common cause of cirrhosis. Tests for hepatitis B and C can determine the presence of these infections and help guide antiviral treatment options. Early detection and management of viral hepatitis are crucial for preventing further liver damage and slowing the progression of cirrhosis. Furthermore, serological tests can identify autoimmune liver diseases, such as autoimmune hepatitis, which may require different management strategies than those used for viral causes of cirrhosis.

In addition to these routine laboratory tests, imaging studies such as ultrasound, CT scans, or MRI may be employed to assess liver structure and detect complications related to cirrhosis, such as portal hypertension or liver tumors. Combining laboratory tests with imaging studies provides a comprehensive picture of liver health and allows for more informed decision-making regarding treatment approaches. Regular follow-up and testing are essential components of managing liver cirrhosis effectively, ensuring that any complications are identified and addressed promptly.

Imaging Studies

Imaging studies play a crucial role in the diagnosis and management of liver cirrhosis. These non-invasive techniques provide valuable information about the liver's structure and function, helping healthcare providers assess the severity of the disease, identify complications, and guide treatment decisions. Common imaging modalities include ultrasound, computed tomography (CT), and magnetic resonance imaging (MRI), each offering distinct advantages and limitations.

Understanding how these studies work and what they can reveal is essential for those managing liver cirrhosis.

Ultrasound is often the first imaging study performed in patients suspected of having liver cirrhosis. This technique uses sound waves to create images of the liver and surrounding structures. It is widely available, cost-effective, and does not involve radiation, making it a safe choice for repeated assessments. Ultrasound can help identify changes in liver size, texture, and blood flow, as well as detect complications like ascites and portal hypertension. Additionally, it can be used to guide procedures such as paracentesis, where fluid is drained from the abdomen.

Computed tomography (CT) scans provide more detailed images than ultrasound and can help identify liver lesions, tumors, or other abnormalities that may arise due to cirrhosis. A CT scan is particularly useful for evaluating the liver's vascular structures and detecting complications such as hepatic encephalopathy or varices.

However, CT scans involve exposure to ionizing radiation and may require the use of contrast agents, which can pose risks for patients with compromised liver function. Therefore, the decision to use CT imaging should be carefully considered based on the individual patient's condition.

Magnetic resonance imaging (MRI) is another advanced imaging modality that offers high-resolution images without radiation exposure. MRI is particularly beneficial in evaluating liver fibrosis and distinguishing between different types of liver lesions. It can also assess blood flow and detect early signs of liver cancer, a common concern in patients with cirrhosis. While MRI is more expensive and less accessible than ultrasound or CT, it provides valuable insights that can influence management strategies and enhance patient care.

In managing liver cirrhosis, the choice of imaging study often depends on the clinical scenario, patient history, and specific questions that need answering. Regular imaging assessments are essential for monitoring disease progression and detecting complications early, which can significantly impact treatment outcomes.

For patients and caregivers, understanding the role of these imaging studies can empower them to engage more actively in discussions with healthcare providers and make informed decisions regarding their care.

Liver Biopsy

Liver biopsy is a medical procedure that involves the removal of a small sample of liver tissue for examination under a microscope. This procedure is crucial in the diagnosis and management of liver cirrhosis, as it provides valuable information about the extent of liver damage, the underlying cause of the cirrhosis, and the presence of any coexisting liver diseases. By obtaining a precise assessment of liver condition, healthcare providers can tailor treatment plans and monitor disease progression more effectively.

There are several methods for performing a liver biopsy, with the most common being percutaneous biopsy, where a thin needle is inserted through the skin into the liver. This procedure is usually guided by ultrasound to ensure accuracy and minimize complications.

Alternatively, a transjugular liver biopsy can be performed, particularly in patients with severe liver disease or when there are concerns about bleeding. In this method, the biopsy needle is threaded through the jugular vein in the neck to reach the liver. Each technique has its indications, benefits, and risks that need to be carefully considered before proceeding.

The decision to perform a liver biopsy is typically based on a combination of clinical factors, laboratory tests, and imaging studies. Patients presenting with elevated liver enzymes, abnormal imaging results, or those with a history of liver disease may be candidates for this procedure. It is important for patients to understand the reasons for the biopsy and the potential outcomes. In some cases, a biopsy may reveal the cause of liver damage, such as viral hepatitis, alcohol-related liver disease, or fatty liver disease, which can significantly influence the management approach.

After the biopsy, patients may experience some discomfort at the biopsy site, but serious complications are rare. Common side effects include pain, bleeding, and infection, but risks are minimized through proper patient selection and technique.

Healthcare providers typically monitor patients for a short period post-procedure to ensure stability. Results from the biopsy are usually available within a few days, and these findings are critical in determining the severity of liver cirrhosis and guiding further management strategies.

In summary, a liver biopsy plays a pivotal role in the effective management of liver cirrhosis. By providing essential diagnostic information, it helps in understanding the underlying causes and guiding treatment decisions. Patients should engage in open discussions with their healthcare providers regarding the necessity, risks, and benefits of the procedure. With the right management plan based on biopsy results, individuals with liver cirrhosis can achieve better health outcomes and improved quality of life.

How To Manage Liver Cirrhosis

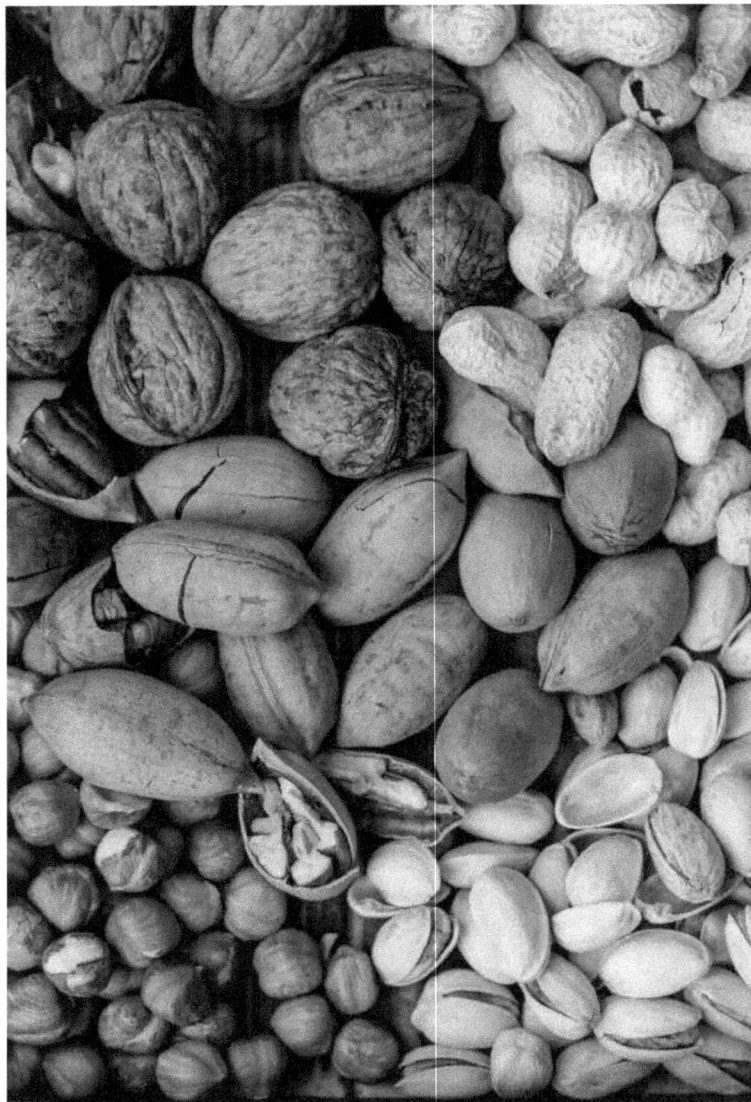

A Comprehensive Guide

Chapter 3

Treatment Options for Liver Cirrhosis

Lifestyle Changes

Lifestyle changes play a crucial role in managing liver cirrhosis and can significantly impact the overall well-being of individuals diagnosed with this condition. The liver is a vital organ responsible for various functions, including detoxification, metabolism, and nutrient storage.

When faced with cirrhosis, it is essential to implement lifestyle modifications that support liver health and prevent further damage. This subchapter outlines several key areas in which individuals can make adjustments to their daily routines.

Diet is one of the most significant aspects of lifestyle change for those managing liver cirrhosis. A balanced diet that emphasizes whole foods, such as fruits, vegetables, whole grains, and lean proteins, is essential. Reducing sodium intake is particularly important, as it can help prevent fluid retention, a common problem in cirrhosis. Individuals should also limit their consumption of processed foods, which often contain high levels of salt and unhealthy fats. Staying well-hydrated by drinking plenty of water can further support liver function, facilitating the removal of toxins from the body.

Physical activity is another vital component of managing liver cirrhosis. Regular exercise can improve overall health, enhance mood, and promote weight management. Low-impact activities, such as walking, swimming, or yoga, are often recommended for individuals with liver issues, as they can be easier on the body while still providing significant benefits. It is essential, however, for individuals to consult with their healthcare provider before starting a new exercise regimen, as they can provide tailored recommendations based on the individual's specific health status.

Alcohol consumption must be completely avoided by anyone managing liver cirrhosis, as it can exacerbate liver damage and complicate the condition further. Even small amounts of alcohol can be detrimental, making complete abstinence critical for individuals with liver issues. Additionally, it is important to be cautious with over-the-counter medications and supplements, as some can be harmful to the liver. Consulting with a healthcare professional before taking any new medications is advisable to ensure safety and compatibility with existing treatments.

Finally, addressing mental health is an often-overlooked aspect of managing liver cirrhosis. The diagnosis of a chronic illness can lead to feelings of anxiety, depression, or isolation. Engaging in support groups or seeking counseling can provide emotional support and coping strategies. Mindfulness practices, such as meditation and deep-breathing exercises, can also help manage stress levels. By focusing on both physical and mental well-being, individuals with liver cirrhosis can create a holistic approach to managing their condition and improving their quality of life.

Medications

Medications play a crucial role in the management of liver cirrhosis, addressing both the underlying causes and the complications that arise from this condition. Patients often require a tailored approach to their medication regimen, depending on the specific etiology of their cirrhosis, such as viral hepatitis, alcohol-related liver disease, or non-alcoholic fatty liver disease. It is essential for patients and caregivers to work closely with healthcare providers to develop a comprehensive plan that considers individual health profiles, potential drug interactions, or presence of other medical conditions.

One of the primary classes of medications used in the management of liver cirrhosis includes antiviral agents for patients with viral hepatitis. These medications help to suppress the replication of the hepatitis virus, reducing liver inflammation and preventing further damage. Common antiviral medications include tenofovir and entecavir for hepatitis B, as well as direct-acting antivirals like sofosbuvir and ledipasvir for hepatitis C. Successful treatment of the underlying viral infection can halt the progression of cirrhosis and improve liver function.

For patients experiencing complications of cirrhosis, such as ascites or hepatic encephalopathy, additional medications may be necessary. Diuretics, such as spironolactone and furosemide, are often prescribed to help manage fluid retention associated with ascites. These medications encourage the kidneys to excrete excess sodium and water, thereby alleviating swelling and discomfort. On the other hand, lactulose and rifaximin are commonly used to treat hepatic encephalopathy, a condition characterized by confusion and altered mental status due to the accumulation of toxins in the bloodstream. These medications work by reducing the levels of ammonia and other harmful substances in the body.

Patients with liver cirrhosis may also require medications to manage portal hypertension, a common complication of the disease. Non-selective beta-blockers, such as propranolol, are frequently prescribed to reduce the risk of variceal bleeding by lowering portal pressure. In some cases, patients may be referred for procedures like endoscopic variceal ligation or transjugular intrahepatic portosystemic shunt (TIPS) in conjunction with medication to manage this complication effectively.

Regular monitoring and adjustment of medications are essential to ensure optimal management of portal hypertension and to prevent serious complications.

It is important for patients and their caregivers to understand the significance of adhering to prescribed medication regimens while being aware of potential side effects. Regular follow-up appointments with healthcare providers are critical for monitoring liver function tests and adjusting medications as needed. Patients should also be educated on recognizing and reporting any adverse effects or changes in their condition promptly. Open communication with healthcare professionals fosters a collaborative approach to managing liver cirrhosis and enhances the overall quality of care.

Surgical Treatments

Surgical treatments for liver cirrhosis are considered when the disease has progressed to a point where non-surgical interventions are insufficient. These procedures aim to alleviate symptoms, manage complications, and improve the quality of life for patients.

Common surgical options include shunt procedures, liver resection, and liver transplantation. Each option has specific indications, risks, and potential benefits that must be carefully evaluated by healthcare professionals in collaboration with patients and their families.

One of the primary surgical interventions for patients with cirrhosis is the creation of a portosystemic shunt. This procedure helps to reduce portal hypertension, a common complication of cirrhosis characterized by increased blood pressure in the portal vein. By redirecting blood flow away from the liver, shunt procedures can alleviate symptoms such as variceal bleeding and ascites. However, these interventions are not without risks, as they can lead to hepatic encephalopathy, a serious condition caused by the accumulation of toxins in the brain due to compromised liver function.

Liver resection, or partial hepatectomy, may be considered for patients with localized liver tumors or complications arising from cirrhosis. In carefully selected cases where the remaining liver tissue is healthy and functioning well, resection can provide significant survival benefits.

However, this procedure requires a thorough assessment of liver function and overall health, as patients with advanced cirrhosis may not tolerate major surgery well. The potential for postoperative liver failure must be weighed against the benefits of removing tumor masses or diseased liver tissue.

Liver transplantation is the most definitive surgical treatment for end-stage liver cirrhosis. It involves the complete removal of the diseased liver and replacement with a healthy liver from a donor. This option is reserved for patients who meet specific criteria, including the severity of liver disease and the absence of contraindications such as active infections or certain cancers. Transplantation offers the possibility of a cure for liver cirrhosis, but it requires lifelong immunosuppressive therapy to prevent organ rejection and comes with its own set of risks and complications.

In conclusion, surgical treatments for liver cirrhosis can provide significant benefits, but they are not suitable for everyone. A multidisciplinary approach involving hepatologists, surgeons, and other specialists is essential for determining the best course of action for each patient.

Ongoing monitoring and follow-up care are crucial to address any complications that may arise from surgical interventions and to ensure optimal management of liver cirrhosis. Engaging with healthcare providers to explore all available options is vital for patients seeking to improve their health outcomes in the context of this chronic disease.

Liver Transplantation

Liver transplantation is a critical intervention for patients suffering from end-stage liver disease, including those with cirrhosis. Cirrhosis can result from various causes, including chronic alcohol consumption, viral hepatitis, and non-alcoholic fatty liver disease. When the liver becomes severely damaged and no longer functions properly, a transplant may become the only viable option for restoring health and prolonging life.

Understanding the transplantation process, eligibility criteria, and post-operative care is essential for individuals managing liver cirrhosis and their families.

Eligibility for liver transplantation involves comprehensive evaluation by a specialized medical team. This assessment includes a thorough review of the patient's medical history, liver function tests, imaging studies, and psychological evaluation. Patients must demonstrate a willingness to adhere to post-transplant care, including lifelong immunosuppressive therapy to prevent organ rejection.

Additionally, factors such as age, overall health, and the presence of other medical conditions will influence a patient's suitability for transplantation. As the waiting list for donor organs can be extensive, timely evaluation and management are crucial for those with cirrhosis.

Once a patient is deemed eligible, they will be placed on a transplant waiting list. During this time, it is vital for patients to maintain regular follow-ups with their healthcare providers and to manage any complications related to their liver disease. Lifestyle modifications, such as maintaining a healthy diet, avoiding alcohol, and managing comorbidities, play a significant role in preparing for surgery.

It is also important for patients and their families to understand the emotional and psychological challenges associated with waiting for a transplant, as the uncertainty and fear can be overwhelming.

The transplantation procedure itself typically involves the surgical removal of the diseased liver and replacement with a healthy liver from a deceased or living donor. This complex surgery requires a high level of skill and precision, and patients can expect a hospital stay of several days to weeks, depending on their recovery progress. Post-operative care is critical for the success of the transplant. Patients will need to adhere to a strict regimen of medications to prevent rejection, monitor liver function regularly, and attend follow-up appointments to ensure optimal recovery.

While liver transplantation can dramatically improve quality of life and survival rates for those with cirrhosis, it is not without risks and complications. Post-transplant patients may face challenges such as infections, organ rejection, and complications related to long-term immunosuppressive therapy.

Therefore, ongoing education about self-management strategies, the importance of adherence to medication regimens, and regular health monitoring is essential for long-term success. By understanding the intricacies of liver transplantation, individuals managing liver cirrhosis can make informed decisions and actively participate in their care journey.

How To Manage Liver Cirrhosis

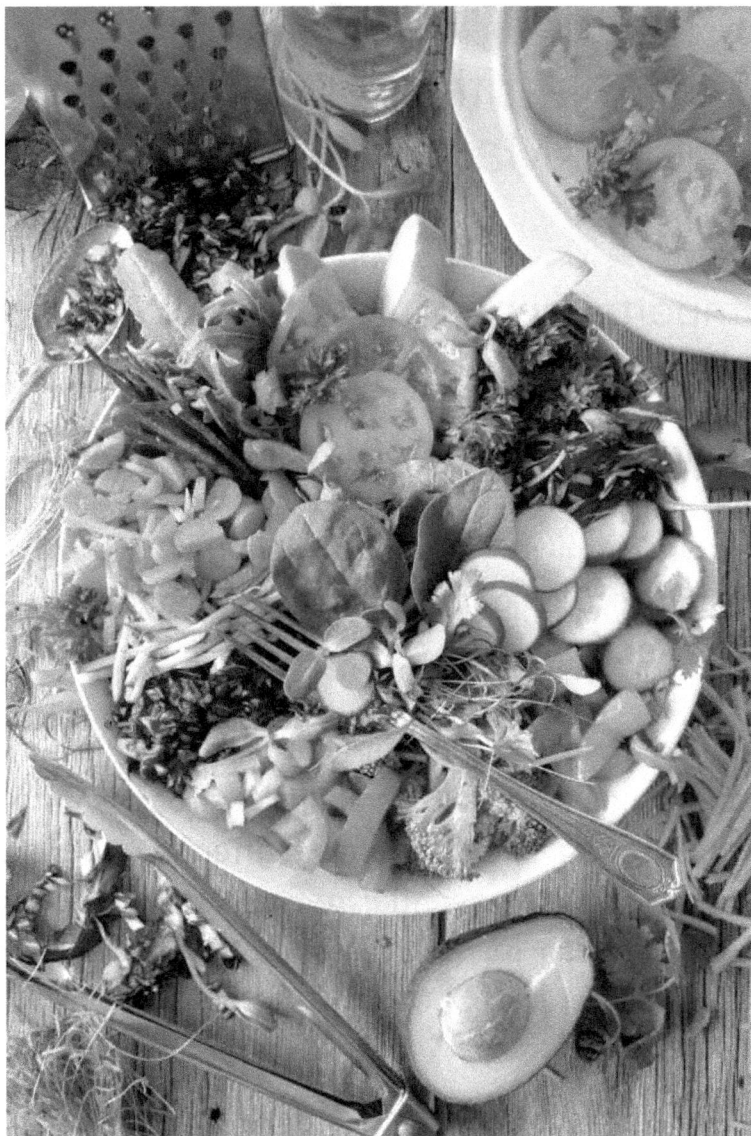

Chapter 4

Nutrition and Diet Management

Importance of Nutrition in Liver Health

Nutrition plays a pivotal role in maintaining liver health, especially for individuals managing liver cirrhosis. The liver is responsible for a myriad of functions, including detoxification, metabolism, and nutrient storage.

When liver function is compromised, as in the case of cirrhosis, the body's ability to process nutrients effectively can be severely affected. Adequate nutrition becomes essential not only to support liver function but also to mitigate symptoms and improve overall quality of life.

A well-balanced diet rich in essential nutrients can help slow the progression of liver disease. Protein intake is particularly important, as it aids in the repair and regeneration of liver tissues. However, it is crucial to choose high-quality protein sources, such as lean meats, fish, eggs, legumes, and dairy products, to ensure that the liver is not overwhelmed by excessive nitrogen from protein metabolism. Additionally, managing protein intake is vital for those experiencing hepatic encephalopathy, where the liver is unable to adequately process ammonia, a byproduct of protein breakdown.

The importance of vitamins and minerals cannot be overstated in the context of liver health. Vitamins A, D, E, and K, along with B-complex vitamins, play significant roles in liver function and overall metabolic processes. Antioxidants found in fruits and vegetables can help combat oxidative stress, which is often elevated in individuals with liver cirrhosis. Incorporating a variety of colorful produce into the diet can provide these essential nutrients while also enhancing the immune system and reducing inflammation.

Healthy fats are another critical component of a liver-friendly diet. Omega-3 fatty acids, found in fatty fish, walnuts, and flaxseeds, have been shown to possess anti-inflammatory properties that may benefit those with liver disease.

It is important to avoid trans fats and limit saturated fats, which can exacerbate liver damage and contribute to weight gain, further complicating cirrhosis management. Instead, focusing on unsaturated fats can promote better liver health and improved metabolic function.

Lastly, hydration plays a fundamental role in maintaining liver health. Adequate fluid intake helps the liver to flush out toxins and supports overall metabolic processes. Individuals managing liver cirrhosis should aim to drink plenty of water while being mindful of electrolyte balance, especially if experiencing complications such as ascites. By prioritizing nutrition and making informed dietary choices, individuals with liver cirrhosis can significantly enhance their liver health and improve their overall well-being.

Recommended Diet for Liver Cirrhosis

A recommended diet for managing liver cirrhosis is critical to slowing the progression of the disease and improving overall health. Individuals with cirrhosis must prioritize a balanced diet that supports liver function while minimizing the intake of harmful substances.

This involves focusing on whole, nutrient-dense foods that provide essential vitamins and minerals, helping to fortify the liver against further damage. It is important to consult with a healthcare provider or a registered dietitian to create a personalized eating plan tailored to individual needs and health conditions.

Protein intake is particularly important for individuals with liver cirrhosis, as it helps in tissue repair and the production of essential enzymes. However, it is crucial to choose high-quality protein sources. Lean meats, fish, eggs, legumes, and low-fat dairy products are excellent options.

For those who are experiencing complications like hepatic encephalopathy, a condition that can arise from liver dysfunction, it may be necessary to adjust protein intake to manage ammonia levels in the blood. This requires careful monitoring and professional guidance to ensure nutritional needs are met without exacerbating symptoms.

In addition to protein, a focus on complex carbohydrates is vital. Whole grains, fruits, and vegetables provide necessary energy and fiber, which can aid digestion and prevent constipation, a common issue for those with liver cirrhosis. Foods rich in antioxidants, such as berries, leafy greens, and nuts, can help neutralize free radicals and support overall liver health. Staying hydrated is also essential; therefore, individuals should aim to drink plenty of water throughout the day while being cautious with fluid intake if they experience fluid retention.

Limiting sodium intake is another critical aspect of dietary management for liver cirrhosis. Excessive sodium can lead to fluid retention and swelling, which can worsen symptoms.

It is advisable to avoid processed foods, canned goods, and salty snacks, opting instead for fresh ingredients and herbs for flavoring. Additionally, individuals should be mindful of their fat intake, focusing on healthy fats from sources like avocados, nuts, and olive oil while minimizing saturated and trans fats found in fried and processed foods.

Lastly, it is essential to avoid alcohol entirely, as it can further damage the liver and accelerate the progression of cirrhosis. Implementing a diet rich in nutrients while avoiding harmful substances can significantly impact the quality of life for those living with cirrhosis. Regular consultations with healthcare professionals can help individuals navigate their dietary choices, ensuring they receive the necessary support and adjustments as their condition evolves.

Foods to Avoid

When managing liver cirrhosis, understanding which foods to avoid is crucial for maintaining health and mitigating symptoms. Certain foods can exacerbate liver damage and lead to complications.

A primary category to avoid is high-sodium foods, which can contribute to fluid retention and increase the risk of edema and ascites. Processed foods, canned soups, and fast food often contain excessive salt, making it essential to read nutrition labels carefully and opt for low-sodium alternatives.

Another group of foods that should be limited is those high in saturated fats and trans fats. These unhealthy fats can worsen liver inflammation and impede its ability to function properly. Foods such as fatty cuts of meat, full-fat dairy products, and fried foods are common culprits. Instead, individuals should focus on healthier fat sources, such as olive oil, avocados, and nuts, which can provide necessary nutrients without overwhelming the liver.

Refined carbohydrates and added sugars also pose significant risks for those with liver cirrhosis. Foods like white bread, pastries, and sugary beverages can lead to insulin resistance and increased fat accumulation in the liver, exacerbating the condition. It is advisable to choose whole grains, fruits, and vegetables instead, as they provide fiber and essential nutrients that support overall liver health.

Alcohol is perhaps the most well-known substance to avoid in managing liver cirrhosis. Even small amounts can lead to further liver damage and increase the risk of complications. Individuals with liver cirrhosis should completely abstain from alcohol to prevent worsening their condition.

It is essential for patients to communicate with healthcare providers about the importance of this abstinence and seek support if needed.

Lastly, certain herbal supplements and over-the-counter medications can be harmful to the liver and should be avoided. Products containing high doses of vitamin A, for example, can lead to toxicity. Additionally, nonsteroidal anti-inflammatory drugs (NSAIDs) and acetaminophen can cause liver strain if used excessively.

Consulting with a healthcare professional before taking any new medications or supplements is vital for safety and effective liver management.

Managing Fluid Intake

Managing fluid intake is a crucial aspect of caring for individuals with liver cirrhosis. The liver plays a vital role in fluid balance, and when it becomes compromised, fluid retention can occur, leading to complications such as ascites and edema. Therefore, it is essential to understand how to regulate fluid consumption effectively to minimize these risks while ensuring adequate hydration.

Patients with liver cirrhosis often need to monitor their fluid intake closely. This typically involves restricting the amount of fluid consumed daily, particularly in the presence of ascites or swelling. The specific fluid limit can vary depending on the severity of the liver disease and the patient's overall health.

Healthcare providers often recommend a fluid intake of around 1 to 1.5 liters per day, but individual needs may differ. Regular consultations with a healthcare professional can help tailor these recommendations to meet personal health goals.

Alongside limiting fluid intake, it is important to focus on the quality of fluids consumed. Opting for low-sodium options is critical, as high sodium levels can exacerbate fluid retention. This includes being mindful of not just table salt, but also processed foods and beverages that may contain hidden sodium.

Additionally, incorporating electrolyte-rich drinks can help maintain hydration without contributing to fluid overload. Patients should consider discussing suitable beverage options with their healthcare team to ensure they are making healthy choices.

Monitoring fluid output is equally important in managing fluid intake. Keeping track of urine output can provide insight into fluid balance and kidney function. Patients should be encouraged to maintain a daily log of their fluid intake and output, which can be shared with their healthcare provider during routine check-ups. This practice not only fosters accountability but also serves as a valuable tool for healthcare professionals to assess the patient's condition and adjust care plans as necessary.

Lastly, understanding the signs of fluid imbalance is crucial for timely intervention. Symptoms such as sudden weight gain, abdominal distension, swelling in the legs, or shortness of breath can indicate fluid overload. Patients and their caregivers should be educated on these warning signs and encouraged to communicate any concerns with their healthcare team promptly. By actively managing fluid intake and being vigilant about changes in body condition, individuals with liver cirrhosis can significantly improve their quality of life and reduce the risk of complications.

How To Manage Liver Cirrhosis

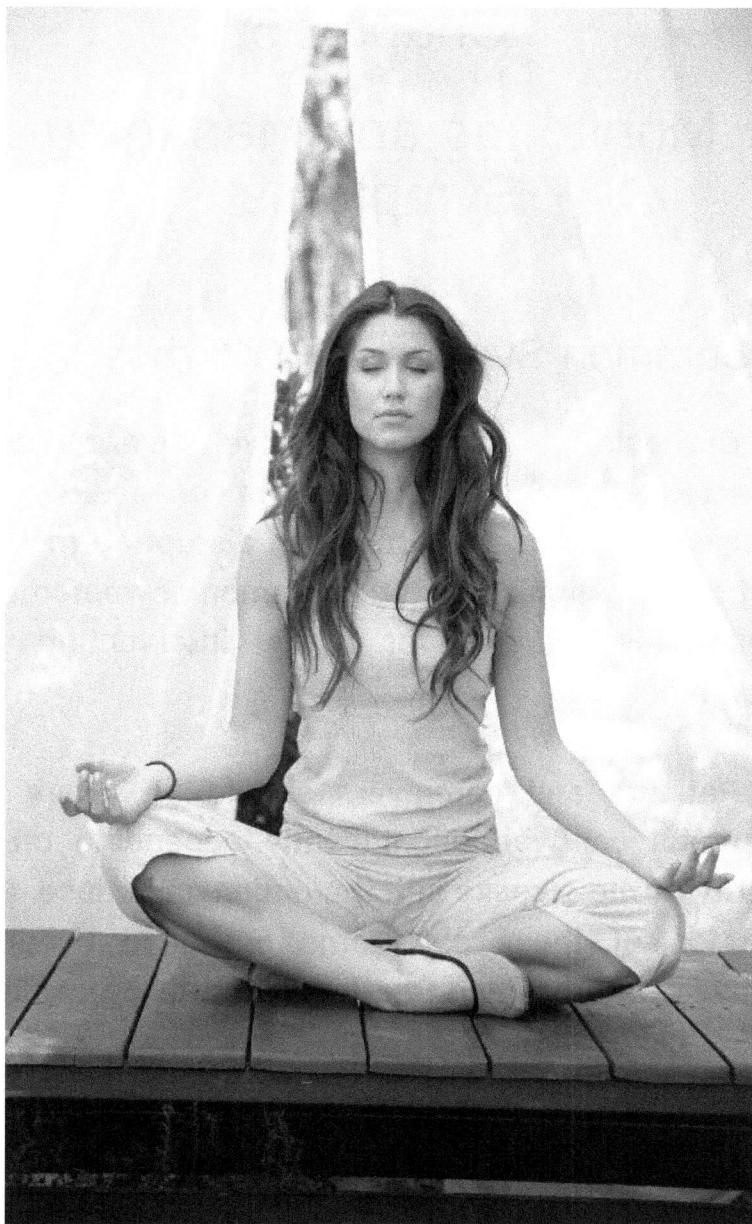

Chapter 5

Monitoring and Managing Symptoms

Common Symptoms of Cirrhosis

Cirrhosis is a progressive liver disease characterized by the replacement of healthy liver tissue with scar tissue, which can disrupt normal liver function. Recognizing the common symptoms of cirrhosis is crucial for early intervention and management.

Patients and caregivers should be aware that symptoms can vary significantly depending on the severity of the disease and the underlying cause. Early detection of these symptoms can lead to timely medical evaluation and treatment, improving quality of life.

One of the most prevalent symptoms of cirrhosis is fatigue, often described as a persistent feeling of tiredness that does not improve with rest. Individuals may find themselves unable to perform daily activities due to a lack of energy. This fatigue can stem from the liver's reduced ability to metabolize nutrients and produce energy. Additionally, the buildup of toxins in the bloodstream due to impaired liver function can contribute to feelings of exhaustion, making it essential to monitor energy levels closely.

Another commonly reported symptom is jaundice, which manifests as a yellowing of the skin and the whites of the eyes. This occurs when the liver is unable to effectively process bilirubin, a byproduct of the breakdown of red blood cells.

As bilirubin accumulates in the body, it leads to discoloration and can also cause itching, adding to the discomfort experienced by individuals with cirrhosis. It is important to note that jaundice may signal worsening liver function and should be evaluated by a healthcare professional promptly.

Fluid retention, or edema, is also a significant symptom of cirrhosis. Patients may notice swelling in the abdomen (ascites) or in the legs and ankles. This occurs due to increased pressure in the blood vessels of the liver, which can lead to leakage of fluid into surrounding tissues. In some cases, this fluid buildup can become severe, necessitating medical intervention. Monitoring weight and abdominal girth can help individuals detect changes early and seek appropriate care.

Other common symptoms include easy bruising and bleeding, due to the liver's role in producing proteins essential for blood clotting. Individuals may notice that cuts take longer to heal or that they develop bruises with minimal trauma. Cognitive changes, often referred to as hepatic encephalopathy, can also occur, leading to confusion, forgetfulness, or changes in mood and behavior. Recognizing these symptoms is vital, as they can indicate the progression of cirrhosis and the need for more intensive management strategies. Understanding these symptoms empowers individuals and their families to take proactive steps in managing liver cirrhosis effectively.

Strategies to Manage Fatigue

Fatigue is a common and often debilitating symptom experienced by individuals with liver cirrhosis. Managing this fatigue effectively is crucial for improving quality of life. One of the primary strategies to combat fatigue involves prioritizing rest and sleep. Establishing a consistent sleep schedule can help regulate the body's internal clock and improve overall energy levels.

Creating a restful environment, free from distractions, can further enhance sleep quality. In addition to nighttime rest, incorporating short naps during the day can provide necessary rejuvenation without interfering with nighttime sleep.

Another effective strategy is to engage in regular, moderate physical activity. While it may seem counterintuitive to exercise when feeling fatigued, light activities such as walking or gentle stretching can actually boost energy levels. Exercise promotes better blood circulation, enhances mood, and can alleviate feelings of tiredness.

It is important to tailor any exercise regimen to the individual's capabilities, gradually increasing intensity as strength improves. Consulting with a healthcare provider or a physical therapist can provide personalized guidance on safe and effective exercise options.

Nutrition plays a pivotal role in managing fatigue associated with liver cirrhosis. A balanced diet rich in vitamins, minerals, and proteins can significantly impact energy levels. It is advisable to focus on whole foods, including fruits, vegetables, whole grains, and lean proteins while avoiding processed foods high in sugars and unhealthy fats.

Staying well-hydrated is equally important, as dehydration can exacerbate feelings of fatigue. Patients should work with a nutritionist specialized in liver health to develop meal plans that support their specific needs and promote overall well-being.

Mental health management is an often-overlooked aspect of combating fatigue. Stress, anxiety, and depression can contribute significantly to feelings of tiredness.

Implementing stress-reduction techniques such as mindfulness, meditation, or yoga can enhance mental clarity and emotional resilience. Support groups or counseling can also provide valuable outlets for sharing experiences and receiving encouragement from others facing similar challenges. Prioritizing mental health is essential not only for managing fatigue but also for fostering a more positive outlook on living with cirrhosis.

Finally, medication management should be closely monitored to address fatigue effectively. Some medications prescribed for liver cirrhosis may contribute to feelings of tiredness. It is crucial for individuals to communicate openly with their healthcare providers about any side effects they experience. Adjustments in medication or dosages can often alleviate fatigue.

Additionally, exploring supplements or alternative therapies under professional guidance may provide additional relief. A comprehensive approach that encompasses rest, physical activity, nutrition, mental health, and medication management is key to effectively managing fatigue in those living with liver cirrhosis.

Handling Jaundice

Handling jaundice in the context of liver cirrhosis requires a thorough understanding of its causes, symptoms, and management strategies. Jaundice, characterized by the yellowing of the skin and eyes, occurs when there is an accumulation of bilirubin in the blood. This condition is often indicative of underlying liver dysfunction, making it a significant concern for individuals with cirrhosis. Effective management begins with recognizing the signs of jaundice and understanding its implications for overall health.

The first step in handling jaundice is to identify its underlying cause, which can vary widely in patients with liver cirrhosis. In many cases, jaundice is a result of the liver's inability to process and excrete bilirubin due to its damaged state. Patients should undergo diagnostic tests, such as blood tests and imaging studies, to determine the severity of liver dysfunction and the presence of any complications. Addressing the root cause of jaundice is essential for effective management, whether it involves treating an infection, managing complications, or adjusting medications.

Dietary changes play a crucial role in managing jaundice in individuals with liver cirrhosis. A well-balanced diet that is low in sodium and rich in essential nutrients can support liver function and overall health. It is important for patients to avoid alcohol, as it can exacerbate liver damage and worsen jaundice. Incorporating foods high in antioxidants, such as fruits and vegetables, may help mitigate liver stress and promote healing.

Consulting a registered dietitian with expertise in liver disease can provide tailored dietary recommendations that align with individual health needs.

In addition to dietary management, regular monitoring of bilirubin levels is vital for individuals experiencing jaundice. Healthcare providers typically recommend routine laboratory tests to track changes in bilirubin levels and assess liver function. This monitoring helps in making informed decisions regarding treatment adjustments and interventions. Patients are encouraged to maintain open communication with their healthcare team, reporting any significant changes in symptoms or concerns regarding jaundice.

Finally, supportive therapies can enhance the quality of life for those dealing with jaundice due to liver cirrhosis. This may include medications to manage symptoms such as itching, which is a common complaint among jaundiced individuals. In some cases, more advanced interventions, such as phototherapy or even liver transplantation, may be considered for severe cases. Integrating a holistic approach that encompasses medical treatment, lifestyle modifications, and emotional support can empower patients to manage jaundice effectively and improve their overall well-being in the face of liver cirrhosis.

Addressing Swelling and Ascites

Swelling and ascites are common complications associated with liver cirrhosis, resulting from increased pressure in the portal vein and changes in the body's fluid balance. Ascites refers specifically to the accumulation of fluid in the abdominal cavity, which can cause discomfort and lead to other health issues. Understanding the underlying mechanisms and recognizing the signs of swelling and ascites are vital for effective management.

Regular monitoring and timely interventions can greatly improve the quality of life for individuals with liver cirrhosis.

To address swelling and ascites, it is crucial to adhere to a low-sodium diet. Sodium can exacerbate fluid retention, worsening symptoms associated with ascites. By limiting sodium intake, individuals can help decrease fluid accumulation and reduce swelling. It is advisable to read food labels carefully and avoid processed foods, which often contain high levels of sodium. Cooking at home using fresh ingredients can also aid in maintaining a low-sodium diet. Consulting with a dietitian can provide personalized dietary recommendations tailored to individual needs.

In some cases, diuretics may be prescribed to help the body eliminate excess fluid. Medications like spironolactone or furosemide can promote urine production, thereby reducing swelling and ascites. It is essential to follow the prescribed dosage and monitor for any side effects, such as electrolyte imbalances, which can occur with long-term use. Regular follow-up appointments with healthcare providers can ensure that the effectiveness of the diuretics is evaluated and adjusted as necessary.

For individuals experiencing severe ascites that do not respond to medical management, more invasive procedures may be required. A paracentesis is a common outpatient procedure used to remove excess fluid from the abdominal cavity, providing immediate relief from discomfort. This procedure may need to be repeated periodically, depending on the severity of the ascites. In some cases, a transjugular intrahepatic portosystemic shunt (TIPS) may be considered, which creates a channel within the liver to redirect blood flow and reduce pressure in the portal vein.

Education and self-management play a critical role in managing swelling and ascites. Individuals should be encouraged to monitor their weight daily, as sudden weight gain can indicate fluid retention. Keeping track of dietary intake, fluid consumption, and symptoms can provide valuable information to healthcare providers. Engaging in light physical activity, as tolerated, may also help promote circulation and prevent further complications. By actively participating in their care, individuals can take significant steps towards managing symptoms and improving their overall well-being.

How To Manage Liver Cirrhosis

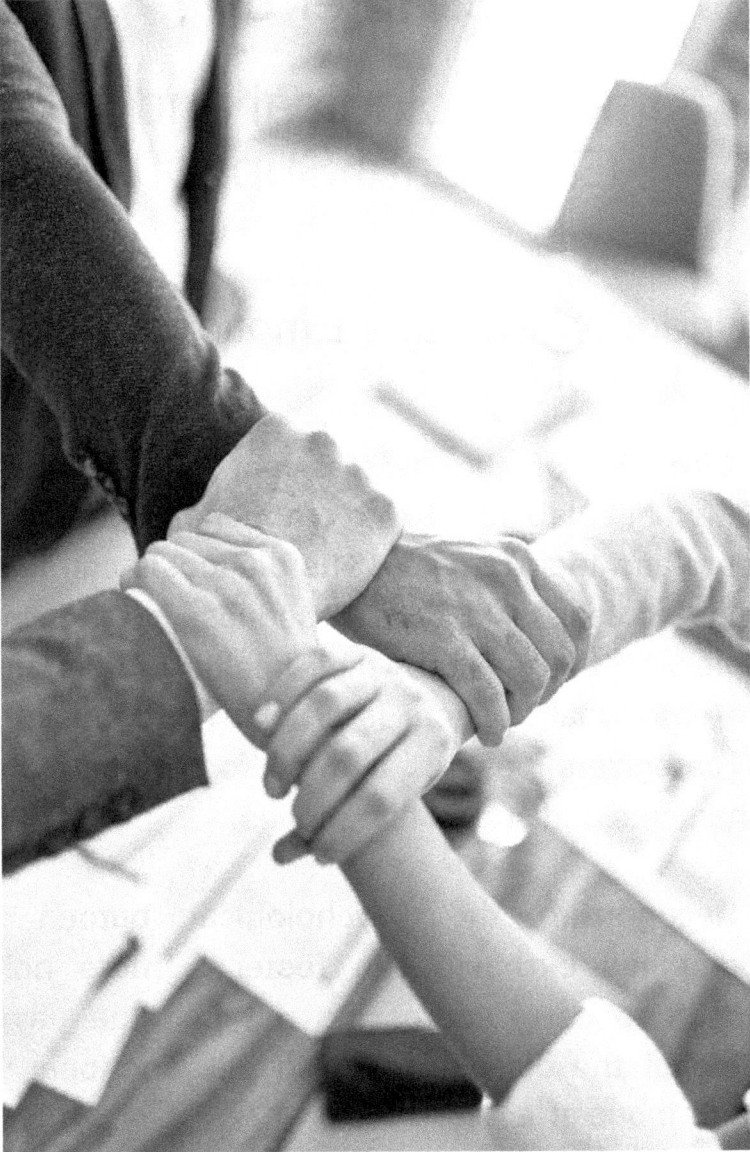

Chapter 6

Psychological and Emotional Support

Understanding the Emotional Impact of Cirrhosis

Cirrhosis of the liver is not only a physical condition but also a profound emotional experience for patients and their families. The diagnosis can lead to feelings of fear, anxiety, and sadness as individuals grapple with the reality of their health. Understanding these emotional impacts is crucial for both patients and caregivers, as it allows for better coping mechanisms and support strategies.

Recognizing the psychological burden that accompanies cirrhosis can foster a more holistic approach to care, addressing not just the physical aspects of the disease but also the emotional well-being of those affected.

Patients often experience a range of emotions, from denial to anger, as they process their diagnosis. Denial may manifest as a reluctance to accept the severity of their condition, leading to potential neglect of necessary lifestyle changes and medical advice. Anger can arise from feelings of helplessness or frustration, particularly if the individual feels that their circumstances are unjust or beyond their control.

It is essential to validate these emotions and encourage open discussions about them. Engaging with a mental health professional can also provide patients with tools to navigate these feelings, enabling them to manage their emotional responses more effectively.

Family members and caregivers are equally impacted by the diagnosis of cirrhosis. They often experience stress and anxiety about their loved one's health, which can lead to feelings of isolation and fear about the future. The caregiver role can be demanding, requiring both physical and emotional support for the patient. It is vital for caregivers to seek support for themselves, whether through support groups or counseling.

This not only helps them cope with their own emotions but also enhances their ability to provide care for the patient. A well-supported caregiver can play a crucial role in the patient's emotional and physical health.

The emotional impact of cirrhosis can also affect interpersonal relationships. Patients may withdraw from social interactions due to feelings of shame or stigma surrounding their condition, which can exacerbate feelings of loneliness and depression. Friends and family may struggle to understand the changes in the patient's behavior, leading to frustration on both sides. Open communication is essential in these situations. Educating loved ones about cirrhosis and its effects can foster empathy and understanding, helping to maintain supportive relationships that are vital to emotional health.

Lastly, incorporating emotional health into the overall management of cirrhosis is essential for comprehensive care. Patients should be encouraged to engage in activities that promote mental well-being, such as mindfulness, exercise, and hobbies that bring joy.

Support groups specifically for those with liver disease can provide a sense of community and shared understanding. By addressing both the physical and emotional aspects of cirrhosis, individuals can create a more balanced approach to their health, ultimately leading to improved outcomes and quality of life.

Coping Strategies for Patients

Coping with liver cirrhosis can be an overwhelming experience for patients and their families. The diagnosis often brings about emotional distress, anxiety, and uncertainty about the future. It is crucial for patients to adopt effective coping strategies to navigate these challenges.

One fundamental approach is establishing a solid support network. This can include family members, friends, and support groups specifically designed for individuals with liver conditions. Engaging with others who share similar experiences can provide emotional relief, practical advice, and a sense of community that is invaluable during difficult times.

Another vital strategy is maintaining open communication with healthcare providers. Patients should feel empowered to ask questions about their condition, treatment options, and lifestyle changes. This transparency fosters a sense of control and understanding, reducing feelings of helplessness. Regular check-ups and follow-ups are essential to monitor the progression of cirrhosis and adjust treatment plans accordingly. Patients are encouraged to document their symptoms, medication side effects, and any changes in their health, which can facilitate more productive discussions with their healthcare team.

Incorporating stress reduction techniques into daily routines can significantly enhance emotional well-being. Mindfulness practices such as meditation, yoga, and deep-breathing exercises help in managing stress and anxiety. These techniques promote relaxation and can improve overall quality of life. Additionally, engaging in light physical activities, as advised by healthcare providers, can boost mood and foster a sense of accomplishment. Patients should aim to find activities that they enjoy, which can serve as an effective distraction from their worries and contribute to their physical health.

Dietary adjustments are also a key component of coping with liver cirrhosis. Patients should work closely with a nutritionist to develop meal plans that are tailored to their specific needs. This often includes reducing sodium intake, avoiding alcohol, and ensuring adequate protein consumption. Educating oneself about foods that support liver health can empower patients and encourage them to make beneficial dietary choices. Cooking at home can also be a therapeutic activity that allows patients to engage with their nutrition actively.

Finally, mental health support should not be overlooked. Many patients with liver cirrhosis experience depression or anxiety, necessitating professional counseling or therapy. Seeking help from mental health professionals can provide coping mechanisms tailored to individual needs, helping patients to process their feelings and adjust to their new reality. Combining these strategies—building a support network, maintaining open communication with healthcare providers, practicing stress reduction techniques, making dietary adjustments, and seeking mental health support—can create a comprehensive framework for coping with liver cirrhosis effectively.

Support for Caregivers

Support for caregivers is a critical component in managing liver cirrhosis effectively. Caregivers often face unique challenges as they navigate the complexities of providing care for individuals with this condition. It is essential for caregivers to have access to resources and support systems that can help them cope with the physical, emotional, and logistical demands of their role. Understanding the nature of liver cirrhosis and its impact on both patients and caregivers can empower those providing care and enhance the quality of life for everyone involved.

One of the most significant challenges caregivers face is the emotional toll of watching a loved one struggle with a chronic illness. Feelings of anxiety, frustration, and sadness are common among caregivers, and it is vital for them to prioritize their own mental health. Engaging in support groups or counseling can provide caregivers with a safe space to share their experiences and feelings. These resources not only offer emotional support but also help caregivers develop coping strategies and connect with others who understand their situation.

Practical support is equally important for caregivers managing the day-to-day tasks associated with liver cirrhosis care. This includes medication management, dietary considerations, and monitoring symptoms. Caregivers should consider collaborating with healthcare professionals to create a comprehensive care plan that outlines specific responsibilities. This collaboration can alleviate some of the burden on caregivers and ensure that they are not navigating the complexities of care alone. Additionally, educational resources tailored to liver cirrhosis can empower caregivers with the knowledge needed to make informed decisions about their loved one's care.

Self-care is a crucial aspect of sustaining the caregiver's ability to provide effective support. Caregivers must remember to take time for themselves, ensuring they engage in activities that promote relaxation and rejuvenation. Simple practices such as regular exercise, maintaining social connections, and pursuing hobbies can significantly improve a caregiver's well-being. By prioritizing their health, caregivers can maintain the energy and resilience needed to support their loved ones through the challenges of liver cirrhosis.

Finally, it is essential for caregivers to communicate openly with their loved ones. Establishing a supportive and understanding dialogue can foster a strong relationship that benefits both the caregiver and the patient. Encouraging patients to express their needs and concerns allows caregivers to provide more tailored support, ultimately leading to better care outcomes. By building a partnership based on trust and transparency, caregivers can better navigate the complexities of liver cirrhosis management, ensuring that both they and their loved ones feel supported throughout the journey.

Professional Counseling Resources

Professional counseling resources play a crucial role in the comprehensive management of liver cirrhosis. Patients and their families often face significant emotional and psychological challenges as they navigate the complexities of the disease. Understanding these resources can provide vital support, helping individuals cope with the stress, anxiety, and lifestyle changes that accompany a diagnosis of cirrhosis.

Accessing professional counseling services can facilitate better emotional well-being and adherence to medical treatment plans.

One of the primary resources available is individual therapy, where patients can engage in one-on-one sessions with a licensed counselor or psychologist. This form of therapy allows individuals to express their feelings, explore coping strategies, and address any mental health concerns that may arise from their condition.

Therapists trained in chronic illness can offer specialized support, helping patients understand their emotions and develop resilience. This personalized approach can empower individuals to manage their disease more effectively.

Group counseling is another valuable resource for those dealing with liver cirrhosis. Support groups provide a safe space for patients to connect with others facing similar challenges. Sharing experiences in a group setting can foster a sense of community and reduce feelings of isolation.

These sessions often include discussions on coping strategies, lifestyle modifications, and emotional support, making them an excellent complement to individual therapy. By hearing others' stories and insights, participants can gain new perspectives and encouragement.

Additionally, many healthcare facilities offer access to social workers who specialize in chronic illnesses. Social workers can assist patients in navigating the healthcare system, providing information about available resources, including financial assistance, transportation services, and educational materials.

They can also help coordinate care among different healthcare providers, ensuring that patients receive comprehensive support. This holistic approach can significantly alleviate stress and improve overall quality of life for individuals managing liver cirrhosis.

Finally, online counseling and teletherapy have emerged as valuable options for those seeking support from the comfort of their homes. With the rise of digital health platforms, patients can access mental health professionals through video calls or messaging, making it easier to fit therapy into their busy lives.

This flexibility is particularly beneficial for individuals with mobility issues or those living in remote areas. By leveraging technology, patients can receive timely support that complements their medical treatment, ultimately enhancing their ability to manage liver cirrhosis effectively.

How To Manage Liver Cirrhosis

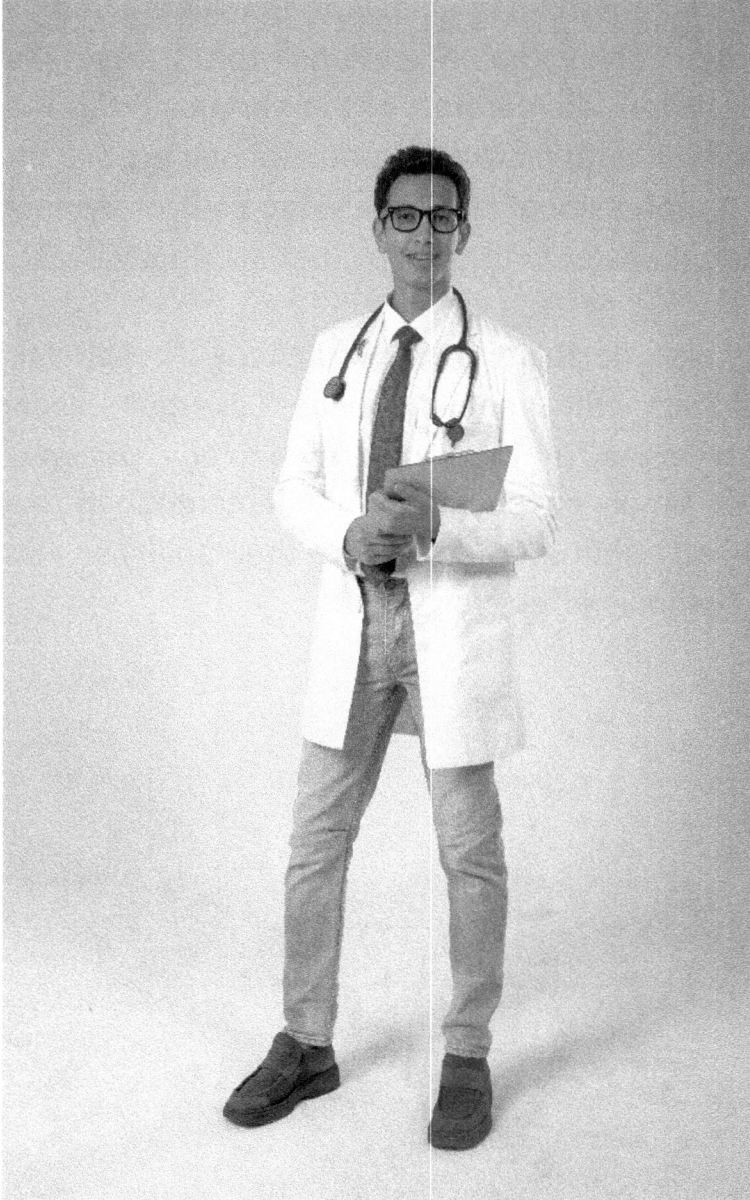

Chapter 7

Regular Medical Care and Follow-up

Importance of Regular Check-ups

Regular check-ups are crucial for individuals managing liver cirrhosis, as they provide an opportunity for healthcare professionals to monitor the progression of the disease and assess liver function. These appointments allow for the evaluation of symptoms, laboratory tests, and imaging studies, which can reveal important changes in liver health.

Early detection of complications, such as liver cancer or portal hypertension, can significantly improve treatment outcomes and quality of life. Regular monitoring also helps in adjusting treatment plans based on the individual's current health status, ensuring that the management of cirrhosis remains effective and responsive to the patient's needs.

During these check-ups, healthcare providers typically perform blood tests to measure liver enzymes, bilirubin levels, and other important markers of liver function. These tests are essential for determining how well the liver is functioning and whether any adjustments in medication or lifestyle are needed. Additionally, imaging studies like ultrasounds or CT scans can help visualize the liver and detect any abnormalities that may require further intervention. By staying proactive with regular appointments, patients can gain valuable insights into their liver health and make informed decisions about their care.

Regular check-ups also offer patients a platform to discuss any new symptoms or concerns with their healthcare team. Symptoms of liver cirrhosis can vary widely, including fatigue, jaundice, and abdominal swelling, and may change over time. Addressing these symptoms promptly can help prevent complications and improve overall health. Furthermore, these appointments provide an opportunity for education about lifestyle modifications that can support liver health, such as dietary changes, exercise, and alcohol avoidance. Engaging in open dialogue with healthcare providers fosters a collaborative approach to managing the condition.

In addition to physical health monitoring, regular check-ups can also address the psychological and emotional aspects of living with liver cirrhosis. Chronic illness can lead to feelings of anxiety, depression, and isolation. Healthcare providers can offer resources and referrals to mental health professionals or support groups, helping patients cope with the emotional challenges of their condition. Regular visits create a routine that not only focuses on physical health but also emphasizes the importance of mental well-being in the management of liver cirrhosis.

Finally, the importance of regular check-ups extends beyond individual care; it contributes to the broader understanding of liver diseases. By participating in routine monitoring, patients contribute valuable data that can help healthcare providers identify trends, develop better treatment protocols, and improve patient outcomes. This collective effort enhances the knowledge base surrounding liver cirrhosis and informs future research and healthcare practices. Through consistent check-ups, individuals with liver cirrhosis can play an active role in their health management while benefiting from the ongoing advancements in medical care.

What to Expect During Appointments

During appointments for managing liver cirrhosis, patients can expect a thorough evaluation of their overall health and liver function. Healthcare providers typically begin with a detailed review of the patient's medical history, including any previous diagnoses, treatments, and lifestyle factors that may impact liver health. Patients should be prepared to discuss their symptoms, such as fatigue, jaundice, or abdominal discomfort, as these details can provide valuable insights for the clinician. It is crucial to be open and honest about alcohol consumption, medication use, and any changes in health, as this information is vital for tailoring an appropriate care plan.

Physical examinations during these appointments often focus on signs of liver disease, such as swelling in the abdomen or legs, changes in skin color, or signs of confusion. The healthcare provider may also check for any complications associated with cirrhosis, such as varices or ascites. Patients should feel comfortable asking questions during this time, as understanding the physical exam findings can help alleviate anxiety and provide clarity about their condition.

It is also important for patients to engage in the discussion about what the physical findings mean for their treatment and overall prognosis.

Laboratory tests play a critical role in managing liver cirrhosis and are commonly conducted during appointments. Blood tests can assess liver function, determine the extent of liver damage, and check for potential complications. Patients should be aware that these tests may include liver function tests, complete blood counts, and tests for viral hepatitis.

Results from these tests can lead to adjustments in medication or changes in treatment strategies. Patients should ask their healthcare provider to explain the significance of the results and how they influence the management plan.

Imaging studies, such as ultrasounds or CT scans, may also be part of the appointment process, especially if there are concerns about liver structure or complications. These non-invasive procedures provide essential information about liver size, blood flow, and the presence of tumors or other abnormalities.

Patients can expect their healthcare provider to discuss the results of these imaging studies and their implications for ongoing management. Understanding the rationale behind these tests can help patients feel more involved in their care and decision-making processes.

Finally, appointments for managing liver cirrhosis are a time for collaborative planning between the patient and the healthcare team. Patients should come prepared with questions and concerns, and they should feel empowered to discuss their preferences regarding treatment options. Health providers will often outline a comprehensive care plan, which may include lifestyle changes, medication management, and monitoring schedules.

Establishing clear communication and setting realistic goals during these appointments can significantly enhance the patient's ability to manage their condition effectively and improve their overall quality of life. Regular follow-ups will be crucial in adjusting the management plan as needed and ensuring that the patient remains on track with their care.

Tracking Progress and Adjusting Treatments

Tracking progress in managing liver cirrhosis is essential for patients and healthcare providers alike. Regular monitoring allows for the assessment of liver function and the effectiveness of treatment plans. Patients should be aware of the key indicators of liver health, such as liver enzyme levels, bilirubin levels, and the presence of complications like ascites or varices. Keeping a detailed record of symptoms and any changes in health status can provide valuable insights during medical appointments, enabling more informed discussions with healthcare professionals.

Routine blood tests play a critical role in tracking the progression of cirrhosis. Healthcare providers typically recommend specific tests to monitor liver function, including alanine aminotransferase (ALT), aspartate aminotransferase (AST), alkaline phosphatase, and albumin levels. Imaging studies such as ultrasound, CT scans, or MRI can also be utilized to evaluate the liver's size, structure, and any potential complications.

Understanding the significance of these tests can empower patients to take an active role in their care, prompting them to seek timely interventions when necessary.

Adjusting treatments based on monitoring results is a crucial aspect of managing cirrhosis effectively. As the disease progresses, treatment strategies may need to be modified to address changing health status or emerging complications.

For instance, if blood tests indicate worsening liver function, a healthcare provider might consider adjusting medications, exploring alternative therapies, or recommending lifestyle changes such as dietary modifications or increased physical activity. Staying engaged with the treatment process and being open to adjustments is vital for optimizing health outcomes.

Communication with healthcare providers is essential when tracking progress and adjusting treatments. Patients should feel comfortable discussing their symptoms, concerns, and any side effects they may be experiencing from medications.

Regular follow-up appointments are necessary to allow for ongoing assessment and to ensure that the treatment plan is aligned with the patient's current health status. Building a collaborative relationship with healthcare professionals can foster an environment where patients feel supported and informed about their care options.

In addition to medical monitoring, patients should consider incorporating holistic approaches to track their progress and manage liver cirrhosis. Keeping a journal that details dietary habits, exercise routines, and emotional well-being can provide a comprehensive overview of how lifestyle choices impact overall health.

Engaging with support groups or counseling services can also offer emotional support and practical advice from others facing similar challenges. This multifaceted approach to tracking progress can enhance the management of liver cirrhosis and lead to better health outcomes.

When to Seek Emergency Care

Recognizing when to seek emergency care is crucial for individuals managing liver cirrhosis, as timely intervention can prevent serious complications. Patients should be aware of specific symptoms that warrant immediate medical attention. These include sudden changes in mental status, such as confusion or disorientation, which may indicate hepatic encephalopathy. Additionally, if a patient experiences severe abdominal pain, particularly in the upper right quadrant, it may signal complications like a ruptured varice or liver abscess, necessitating urgent evaluation.

Another critical sign that requires prompt care is the onset of gastrointestinal bleeding, which can manifest as vomiting blood or passing black, tarry stools. These symptoms often indicate variceal bleeding, a serious complication of cirrhosis. Patients should also seek emergency help if they notice significant swelling in the abdomen or legs, which could indicate fluid retention or ascites. Rapid weight gain due to fluid accumulation can lead to discomfort and may require immediate medical management.

Infections pose a significant risk to individuals with liver cirrhosis, and symptoms such as fever, chills, or persistent fatigue should not be overlooked. Patients with cirrhosis have a compromised immune system, making them more susceptible to infections, particularly spontaneous bacterial peritonitis, which can arise from fluid accumulation in the abdomen.

If any signs of infection appear, it is essential to consult a healthcare provider without delay to prevent further complications.

Additionally, any sudden or unexplained changes in urine color, particularly dark urine or pale stools, should prompt an immediate medical consultation. Dark urine may indicate liver dysfunction or bile obstruction, while pale stools could suggest a lack of bile reaching the intestines.

Both conditions can signify worsening liver function and require urgent assessment and intervention to manage potential complications.

Finally, it is critical for patients and caregivers to maintain open communication with healthcare providers regarding any concerning symptoms. Establishing a clear action plan for emergencies can empower individuals to make informed decisions about their health. Understanding when to seek emergency care is a vital aspect of managing liver cirrhosis effectively, ensuring that complications are addressed promptly to maintain health and well-being.

How To Manage Liver Cirrhosis

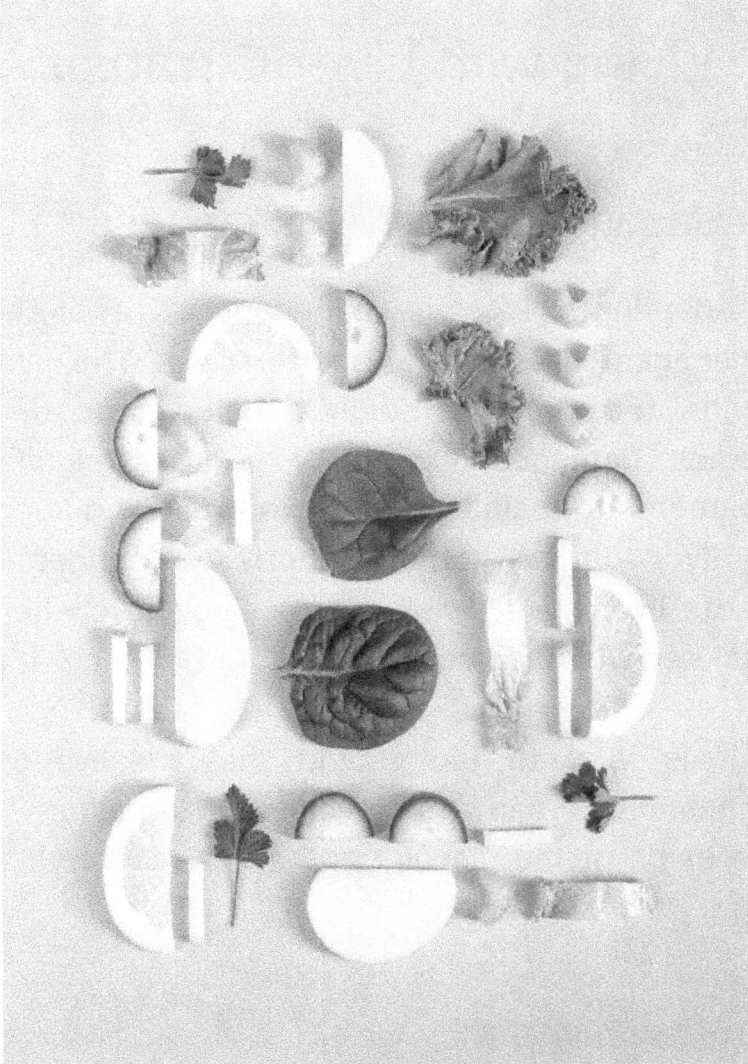

Chapter 8

Living with Liver Cirrhosis

Adapting to Lifestyle Changes

Adapting to lifestyle changes is a crucial aspect of managing liver cirrhosis effectively. The liver is essential for numerous bodily functions, and when it becomes damaged, the body requires significant adjustments to maintain health. Individuals diagnosed with liver cirrhosis must prioritize changes that promote liver health while addressing the challenges associated with their condition.

It is vital to understand that these lifestyle modifications can significantly influence the progression of the disease and enhance overall well-being.

One of the most significant lifestyle changes involves dietary adjustments. A balanced diet that is low in sodium and rich in essential nutrients can help reduce the workload on the liver. This includes incorporating plenty of fruits, vegetables, whole grains, and lean proteins while avoiding processed foods high in salt and sugar.

Patients may also need to limit their intake of alcohol, as even small amounts can exacerbate liver damage. Consulting with a nutritionist can provide tailored dietary recommendations that meet individual health needs and preferences.

Regular physical activity plays a vital role in managing liver cirrhosis. Engaging in moderate exercise can help maintain a healthy weight, improve energy levels, and enhance overall physical health. Activities such as walking, swimming, or gentle yoga can be beneficial, but it is important for individuals to consult with their healthcare provider before starting any new exercise regimen. Establishing a consistent routine can foster a sense of normalcy and empowerment, allowing patients to take an active role in their health management.

In addition to dietary and exercise changes, emotional and mental well-being must also be addressed. Living with liver cirrhosis can lead to feelings of anxiety, depression, or isolation. Establishing a strong support network, whether through family, friends, or support groups, can provide emotional assistance and help individuals cope with the challenges of their condition. Mindfulness practices, such as meditation or deep-breathing exercises, can also serve as effective tools for managing stress and improving mental health.

Lastly, regular medical check-ups and monitoring are essential components of adapting to lifestyle changes. Keeping up with appointments and following healthcare provider recommendations ensures that individuals can track their liver function and make necessary adjustments to their care plan. Staying informed about the latest research and treatment options can also empower patients to make informed decisions regarding their health. By embracing these lifestyle changes and remaining proactive, individuals can successfully manage liver cirrhosis and enhance their quality of life.

Building a Support Network

Building a support network is crucial for individuals managing liver cirrhosis. This condition can be emotionally and physically taxing, making it essential to surround oneself with people who understand the challenges involved. A strong support network can provide encouragement, share valuable resources, and offer practical assistance, which can significantly improve the quality of life for those affected. It is important to recognize that this network can include family, friends, healthcare professionals, and support groups, each playing a unique role in the journey of managing liver cirrhosis.

Family and friends often form the backbone of a support network. They can offer emotional support by being present during difficult times and providing a listening ear. It can be beneficial to communicate openly with loved ones about the condition and its implications. Sharing information about liver cirrhosis helps them understand the situation better, enabling them to provide more targeted support. Encouraging family members to attend medical appointments can also help them grasp the intricacies of the condition and become more involved in care decisions.

Healthcare professionals are another vital component of a support network. This group includes primary care physicians, hepatologists, nutritionists, and mental health counselors. Each professional can contribute specific expertise that is crucial for managing liver cirrhosis effectively. Regular consultations with these experts can ensure that individuals receive up-to-date information on treatment options, dietary recommendations, and mental health resources. Building a rapport with these professionals can facilitate open communication and foster a collaborative approach to care, enhancing overall well-being.

Support groups provide a unique platform for individuals dealing with liver cirrhosis to connect with others facing similar challenges. These groups can be found in various formats, including in-person meetings and online forums. Participating in a support group allows individuals to share experiences, coping strategies, and emotional burdens. Hearing from others who have navigated similar situations can instill hope and resilience, while also reducing feelings of isolation. Support group members often share valuable resources and information that can aid in managing the condition more effectively.

Finally, it's essential to remember that building a support network is an ongoing process. As circumstances change, so may the needs for support. Regularly assessing the effectiveness of the network and making adjustments as necessary can help maintain a strong foundation.

This might involve seeking new connections, whether through local organizations or online communities, to ensure that individuals have access to diverse perspectives and resources. By proactively managing and nurturing a support network, those affected by liver cirrhosis can enhance their coping mechanisms and improve their overall health outcomes.

Planning for the Future

Planning for the future when managing liver cirrhosis is crucial for maintaining health and well-being. Individuals diagnosed with this condition often face uncertainties regarding their health, treatment options, and lifestyle changes.

Therefore, having a strategic plan can help individuals navigate their journey more effectively. This plan should encompass medical management, nutritional considerations, emotional support, and lifestyle adjustments to ensure a holistic approach to care.

Medical management is the cornerstone of planning for the future with liver cirrhosis. Regular consultations with healthcare providers are essential to monitor liver function and overall health. Patients should be proactive in scheduling routine check-ups and tests, such as liver function tests and imaging studies, to assess the progression of the disease.

Additionally, staying informed about potential complications of cirrhosis, including portal hypertension and liver cancer, is vital. It's important for patients to discuss any new symptoms with their healthcare team promptly, as early intervention can significantly improve outcomes.

Nutrition plays a pivotal role in managing liver cirrhosis and should be a key component of future planning. A well-balanced diet tailored to the needs of individuals with liver disease can help prevent malnutrition and support liver function. Patients are often advised to limit salt intake to reduce fluid retention and to consume adequate protein to maintain muscle mass. Consulting a registered dietitian who specializes in liver health can provide personalized nutritional guidance. Additionally, staying hydrated and avoiding alcohol are essential steps in promoting liver health and enhancing quality of life.

Emotional and psychological support should not be overlooked when planning for the future. The diagnosis of liver cirrhosis can lead to feelings of anxiety, depression, or uncertainty. Engaging in support groups or counseling can provide a safe space for expressing feelings and sharing experiences with others facing similar challenges. Building a strong support network, including family and friends, is also vital. Encouraging open communication about fears and concerns regarding the disease can foster a sense of community and reassurance.

Finally, lifestyle adjustments are necessary for effective management of liver cirrhosis. Incorporating regular physical activity tailored to the individual's abilities can enhance physical health and improve mood. Stress management techniques, such as mindfulness, yoga, or meditation, can also contribute to overall well-being. Setting achievable goals related to health and lifestyle can empower individuals to take charge of their condition. By creating a comprehensive plan that addresses medical, nutritional, emotional, and lifestyle factors, individuals can better prepare for the future and enhance their quality of life while living with liver cirrhosis.

Resources and Support Groups

Resources and support groups play a crucial role in managing liver cirrhosis, providing patients and their families with the necessary tools and information to navigate the complexities of the disease. Understanding the available resources can empower patients to take an active role in their care, leading to better health outcomes. Numerous organizations, both national and local, focus on liver health and can provide valuable educational materials, support, and advocacy for those affected by liver cirrhosis.

One of the primary resources for individuals dealing with liver cirrhosis is the American Liver Foundation. This organization offers a wealth of information on liver diseases, including cirrhosis, and provides access to educational programs, webinars, and research updates. Their website contains articles, brochures, and guidelines on managing liver health, dietary recommendations, and potential treatment options. Furthermore, the foundation often hosts events and seminars that can help patients connect with healthcare professionals and other individuals facing similar challenges.

Support groups can also be instrumental in the journey of managing liver cirrhosis. These groups provide a safe space for patients and caregivers to share experiences, discuss coping strategies, and offer emotional support. Many hospitals and clinics offer in-person support groups led by healthcare professionals, while online communities provide a platform for individuals to connect regardless of their geographical location. Participating in these groups can reduce feelings of isolation and foster a sense of belonging among those affected by the disease.

Additionally, healthcare providers play a critical role in guiding patients toward the appropriate resources. Patients should feel encouraged to communicate openly with their doctors about their needs for information and support. Healthcare professionals can recommend local resources, such as nutritionists specializing in liver health or mental health counselors familiar with chronic illness. They can also provide referrals to support groups and educational workshops designed for those with liver cirrhosis.

Finally, patients should utilize digital resources, such as reputable websites and mobile applications that focus on liver health. Many online tools offer symptom tracking, medication reminders, and dietary advice tailored to the needs of those with liver cirrhosis. Social media platforms can also serve as a means to connect with others facing similar struggles, fostering community and shared learning. By leveraging a variety of resources and support groups, individuals managing liver cirrhosis can enhance their quality of life and better navigate their healthcare journey.

How To Manage Liver Cirrhosis

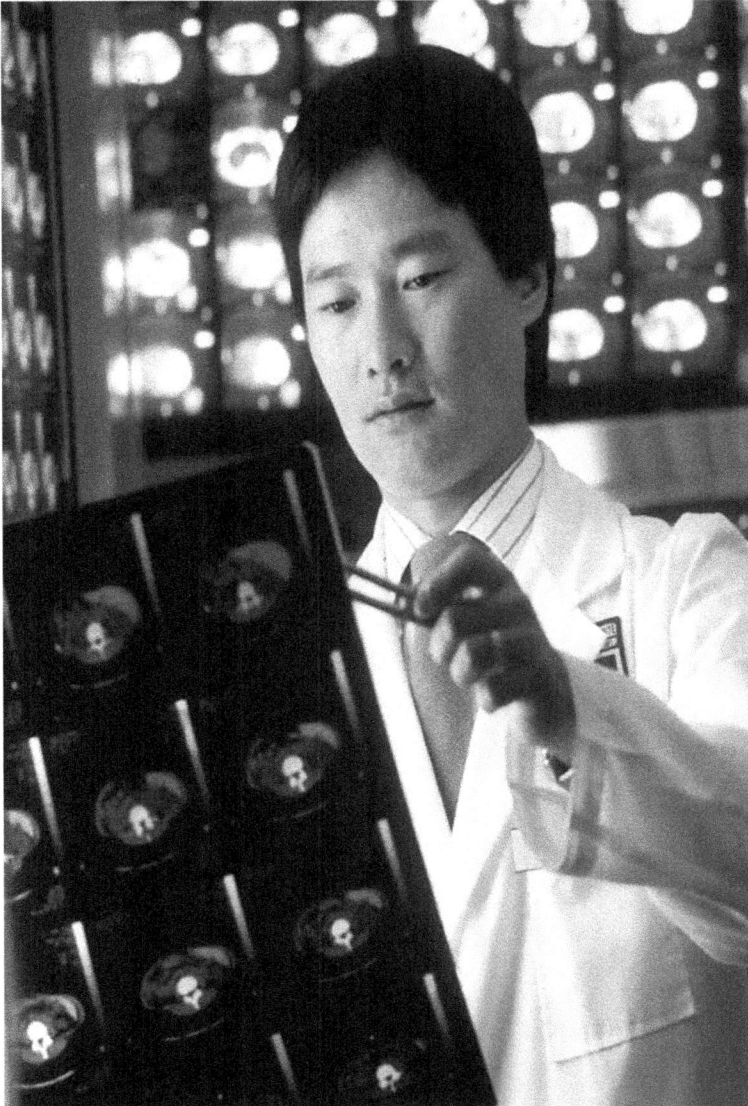

Chapter 9

Prevention and Risk Reduction

Avoiding Alcohol and Drug Use

Avoiding alcohol and drug use is crucial for individuals managing liver cirrhosis. Alcohol, in particular, poses a significant risk to liver health, as it can exacerbate liver damage and accelerate the progression of the disease.

For those already diagnosed with cirrhosis, even small amounts of alcohol can lead to serious complications, including liver failure and increased vulnerability to infections. It is essential to understand that the liver is already compromised, and consuming alcohol can further impair its ability to function effectively.

In addition to alcohol, recreational and illicit drugs can also have detrimental effects on liver health. Many substances are metabolized by the liver, and their use can lead to additional stress on this vital organ.

For individuals with liver cirrhosis, the use of drugs can result in unpredictable reactions, increased toxicity, and a higher likelihood of adverse side effects. It is vital to avoid any substances that could further compromise liver function or interact negatively with prescribed medications.

Education plays a critical role in avoiding alcohol and drug use. Individuals should be informed about the risks associated with substance use and its impact on their overall health.

Attending support groups or therapy can provide valuable resources and coping strategies for those struggling with addiction or the temptation to use substances. Knowledge about the potential consequences of alcohol and drug use can empower individuals to make informed decisions that prioritize their liver health.

Creating a supportive environment is another essential aspect of avoiding substance use. Friends and family members can play a significant role in encouraging healthy habits and providing emotional support. It is beneficial for individuals to communicate their health concerns with loved ones, as this transparency can foster understanding and support. Establishing a network of support can help individuals stay accountable and focused on their journey to manage liver cirrhosis effectively.

Finally, developing healthy coping mechanisms is vital for individuals looking to avoid alcohol and drug use. Engaging in activities such as exercise, mindfulness practices, and hobbies can provide healthy outlets for stress and emotional challenges. By replacing negative habits with positive ones, individuals can improve their overall well-being and reduce the likelihood of turning to substances for relief.

Emphasizing the importance of lifestyle changes and self-care can significantly contribute to better management of liver cirrhosis and promote long-term health.

Vaccinations and Preventive Measures

Vaccinations play a critical role in the management of liver cirrhosis, as individuals with this condition are more susceptible to infections. The immune system may be compromised due to liver dysfunction, making it essential for patients to stay up to date with their vaccinations. Hepatitis A and B vaccinations are particularly important, as these viruses can exacerbate liver disease and lead to further complications. Additionally, the influenza vaccine is recommended annually to help prevent respiratory infections that can stress the liver. Pneumococcal vaccines are also advised, as individuals with cirrhosis are at a higher risk for pneumonia and other respiratory illnesses.

Preventive measures extend beyond vaccinations and include lifestyle modifications that can significantly impact liver health. Maintaining a balanced diet rich in fruits, vegetables, and whole grains supports the immune system and overall health. Staying hydrated is crucial, as it aids in digestion and helps the liver function more efficiently.

Regular physical activity, tailored to the individual's capabilities, can improve circulation and enhance overall well-being. Avoiding alcohol is imperative, as it can further damage an already compromised liver and lead to additional health issues.

Routine medical check-ups and screenings are vital components of preventive care for individuals with liver cirrhosis. Regular monitoring of liver function through blood tests allows healthcare providers to assess the progression of the disease and make necessary adjustments to treatment plans. Patients should also undergo screenings for liver cancer, especially if they have cirrhosis due to hepatitis B or C infections. Early detection of complications can significantly improve outcomes and quality of life for those affected.

In addition to vaccinations and lifestyle adjustments, education plays a crucial role in prevention. Patients and caregivers should be informed about the signs of liver complications and the importance of prompt medical intervention when symptoms arise.

Knowledge about the risks associated with cirrhosis, such as the potential for bleeding or infection, empowers individuals to seek timely care.

Support groups and educational resources can also provide valuable information and foster a sense of community among those managing liver cirrhosis.

Lastly, collaboration with healthcare providers is essential for effective prevention strategies. Open communication about concerns, treatment options, and lifestyle changes can lead to a more personalized approach to care. Patients should feel encouraged to discuss their experiences and ask questions about their health.

A comprehensive care plan that incorporates vaccinations, preventive measures, and regular follow-ups can greatly enhance the quality of life for individuals living with liver cirrhosis and reduce the risk of serious complications.

Managing Comorbidities

Managing comorbidities in patients with liver cirrhosis is an essential aspect of care that significantly impacts overall health outcomes. Comorbidities, or the presence of additional diseases alongside liver cirrhosis, can complicate treatment and exacerbate complications related to liver dysfunction. Common comorbidities associated with liver cirrhosis include diabetes, hypertension, cardiovascular diseases, and renal impairment. Addressing these conditions proactively can improve quality of life and potentially enhance liver function, making it crucial for patients and caregivers to understand the interplay between liver health and these accompanying conditions.

One of the primary comorbidities seen in patients with liver cirrhosis is diabetes, particularly type 2 diabetes. Insulin resistance is frequently observed in individuals with liver disease, which can lead to complications such as hyperglycemia. Effective management of blood sugar levels is vital, requiring a careful selection of medications that do not adversely affect liver health.

Patients should work closely with their healthcare providers to monitor glucose levels and adjust treatment plans as necessary, incorporating lifestyle modifications such as diet and exercise to help manage both diabetes and cirrhosis simultaneously.

Hypertension is another prevalent comorbidity that complicates the management of liver cirrhosis. Cirrhotic patients may experience portal hypertension, which can lead to serious complications such as variceal bleeding. Controlling blood pressure in this population is critical for preventing further complications.

Patients are encouraged to engage in regular monitoring of their blood pressure and to follow prescribed antihypertensive therapies. A low-sodium diet and regular physical activity can also play a significant role in managing hypertension while being mindful of the limitations imposed by liver disease.

Cardiovascular health is a significant concern for patients with liver cirrhosis, as they are at an increased risk of heart disease due to factors such as fluid overload and metabolic disturbances.

Regular cardiovascular assessments are recommended, including monitoring of lipid profiles and heart function. Patients should be informed about the importance of adhering to cardiovascular medications and lifestyle interventions that support heart health, which may include quitting smoking, maintaining a healthy weight, and engaging in moderate exercise, tailored to their abilities and health status.

Finally, renal impairment is a serious comorbidity that can arise in patients with liver cirrhosis, often leading to hepatorenal syndrome, a condition characterized by rapid kidney failure. It is essential for patients to have their renal function monitored regularly through blood work and urine tests.

Preventive measures, such as avoiding nephrotoxic medications and maintaining adequate hydration, can help mitigate the risk of renal complications. By managing comorbidities effectively, patients can enhance their overall health and improve their prognosis, making a comprehensive approach to care in liver cirrhosis vital for better outcomes.

Educating Family and Friends

Educating family and friends about liver cirrhosis is an integral part of managing the condition effectively. When loved ones understand the complexities of cirrhosis, they can provide better emotional and practical support. Begin by explaining what liver cirrhosis is—a late-stage scarring of the liver caused by various factors, including chronic alcohol use, viral infections, and fatty liver disease. This understanding helps demystify the condition and alleviates any misconceptions that may exist regarding its causes and effects.

It is essential to discuss the symptoms and complications associated with liver cirrhosis so that family and friends can recognize warning signs and provide appropriate assistance. Symptoms may include fatigue, jaundice, and abdominal swelling, which can significantly impact daily life. By educating them about these signs, you empower your support network to respond promptly in times of need. It is also beneficial to address common complications such as portal hypertension and liver failure, which may require immediate medical attention.

Involving family and friends in the management plan is crucial for creating a supportive environment. Encourage them to participate in medical appointments or discussions with healthcare providers if the patient is comfortable. This inclusion not only fosters understanding but also enables loved ones to ask questions and clarify doubts.

Additionally, discussing dietary changes and lifestyle modifications, such as avoiding alcohol and maintaining a healthy diet, can help them understand how they can assist in promoting better health outcomes.

Communication is key in educating your support network about the emotional and psychological aspects of living with liver cirrhosis. Patients may experience feelings of anxiety, depression, or isolation as they navigate their diagnosis.

By openly sharing these feelings with family and friends, you promote a culture of empathy and support. Encourage loved ones to engage in conversations about mental health and to be active listeners, which can create a safe space for expressing concerns and fears.

Finally, provide resources that family and friends can reference for further information on liver cirrhosis. This may include reputable websites, support groups, or informational pamphlets from healthcare providers. By equipping them with knowledge, you enhance their ability to contribute positively to your care journey. A well-informed support network can alleviate stress and foster a sense of community, which is invaluable in managing the challenges associated with liver cirrhosis.

How To Manage Liver Cirrhosis

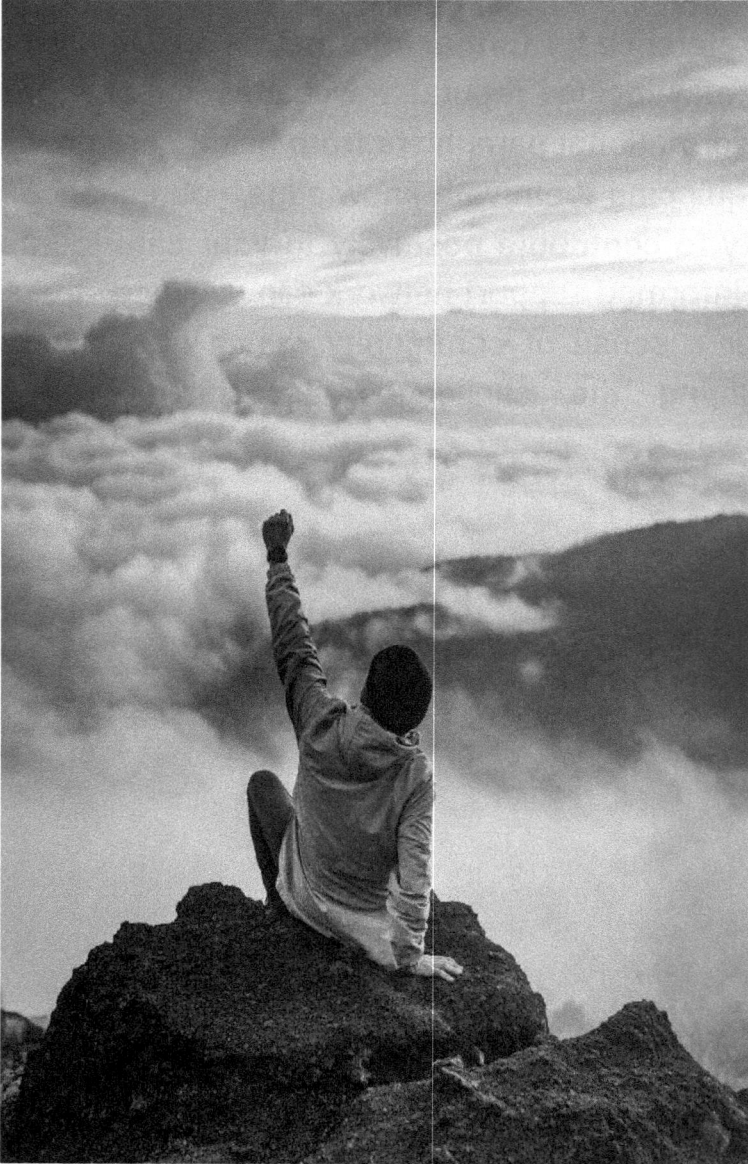

A Comprehensive Guide

Chapter 10

Conclusion and Future Directions

Summary of Key Takeaways

The management of liver cirrhosis requires a multifaceted approach that prioritizes patient education, lifestyle modifications, and regular medical oversight. Understanding the progressive nature of cirrhosis is crucial for individuals affected by the condition.

This liver disease, characterized by the replacement of healthy liver tissue with scar tissue, can lead to severe complications if not managed properly. Key takeaways emphasize the importance of early detection and intervention, which can significantly improve quality of life and prognosis for those living with cirrhosis.

A critical aspect of managing liver cirrhosis is adhering to a well-structured dietary plan. Patients are encouraged to consume a balanced diet rich in fruits, vegetables, whole grains, and lean proteins while limiting sodium intake to manage fluid retention. Staying hydrated is also essential, as it aids in overall liver function. Moreover, individuals should avoid alcohol completely, as it further exacerbates liver damage. Nutrition plays a pivotal role, and consulting with a registered dietitian can provide tailored advice that supports liver health.

Regular medical check-ups and monitoring are indispensable for anyone managing cirrhosis. These appointments allow healthcare providers to track disease progression and adjust treatment plans accordingly. Blood tests, imaging studies, and assessments for complications such as varices or hepatic encephalopathy are standard practices.

Additionally, being vigilant about vaccinations, especially for hepatitis A and B, can help prevent further liver complications. Engaging in open communication with healthcare professionals fosters a collaborative approach to care.

Psychosocial support is another essential component of managing liver cirrhosis. Living with a chronic illness can lead to emotional and mental health challenges. Finding support groups or counseling services can provide a safe space for sharing experiences and coping strategies. Encouraging family involvement can also create a supportive environment, making it easier for patients to adhere to their treatment plans. Mental health is as vital as physical health, and addressing it can lead to better overall outcomes.

Lastly, it is important for patients to be proactive in their self-care routines and to stay informed about their condition. Keeping up with educational resources, attending workshops, and connecting with other individuals facing similar challenges can empower patients. Understanding the implications of cirrhosis, recognizing the symptoms of complications, and knowing when to seek medical attention are vital skills. Through a combination of knowledge, support, and lifestyle adjustments, individuals can take significant steps towards effectively managing liver cirrhosis and improving their overall health and well-being.

Future Research and Developments

Future research and developments in the management of liver cirrhosis are crucial for enhancing patient care and outcomes. As our understanding of liver diseases evolves, innovative therapeutic approaches are being explored. Recent advancements in molecular biology and genetics have opened new avenues for identifying biomarkers that could lead to earlier diagnosis and personalized treatment strategies.

Research is focused on understanding the underlying mechanisms of liver fibrosis and cirrhosis to develop targeted therapies that can halt or even reverse liver damage.

One promising area of research is the application of stem cell therapy in the treatment of liver cirrhosis. Scientists are investigating the potential of stem cells to regenerate damaged liver tissue and restore normal function. Clinical trials are underway to assess the efficacy and safety of these therapies, which could offer hope for patients with advanced liver disease.

Additionally, the use of mesenchymal stem cells, which have immunomodulatory properties, may lead to improved liver function and reduced inflammation in cirrhotic patients.

Another exciting development in the management of liver cirrhosis is the exploration of novel pharmacological agents. Researchers are evaluating new medications that target specific pathways involved in liver fibrosis progression. For instance, antifibrotic agents are being studied to determine their capacity to reduce or reverse liver fibrosis. The results of these studies could have significant implications for the treatment of cirrhosis, providing new options for patients who currently have limited choices.

Technological advancements are also playing a vital role in the future of liver cirrhosis management. Non-invasive imaging techniques, including elastography and advanced MRI methods, are being refined to better assess liver stiffness and fibrosis. These tools can help clinicians monitor disease progression more accurately and tailor treatment plans accordingly.

Furthermore, the integration of artificial intelligence in predictive analytics may assist healthcare providers in identifying patients at high risk for complications, enabling timely interventions.

Finally, patient education and lifestyle modifications remain integral to the management of liver cirrhosis, and future research will likely focus on understanding how these factors influence disease progression and patient outcomes. Studies examining the impact of diet, exercise, and psychosocial support on liver health will provide valuable insights. By combining cutting-edge research with a holistic approach to patient care, the future of managing liver cirrhosis holds promise for improved quality of life and survival rates for those affected by this challenging condition.

Final Thoughts on Living Well with Cirrhosis

Living well with cirrhosis requires a multifaceted approach that encompasses medical care, lifestyle adjustments, and emotional support. Understanding the nature of cirrhosis is essential, as it is a progressive condition resulting from liver damage.

Awareness of the disease and its progression helps patients and caregivers make informed decisions about management strategies. Regular consultations with healthcare professionals can help monitor liver function, assess complications, and adjust treatment plans as necessary, ensuring that individuals are receiving the optimal care needed to maintain their health.

Diet plays a crucial role in managing liver cirrhosis. Patients are often advised to adopt a balanced diet that focuses on nutrient-rich foods while avoiding those that can exacerbate liver damage. Reducing sodium intake is particularly important for those with fluid retention, while protein consumption must be tailored to the individual's needs, especially in cases of hepatic encephalopathy.

Engaging with a nutritionist who specializes in liver diseases can provide personalized dietary guidance and help patients navigate food choices that support liver health and overall well-being.

Physical activity is another vital component of living well with cirrhosis. While exercise may seem daunting, especially for those experiencing fatigue or weakness, even light physical activity can enhance physical strength, improve mood, and support liver function. Tailoring an exercise routine that fits individual capabilities and energy levels is essential. Activities such as walking, stretching, or gentle yoga can be beneficial. Consulting with healthcare providers before starting any new exercise program ensures that activities are safe and suitable for the patient's condition.

Emotional and psychological well-being is often overlooked in the management of chronic illnesses like cirrhosis. The stress of living with a progressive disease can lead to anxiety, depression, and social withdrawal. Seeking support from mental health professionals, joining support groups, or connecting with others who share similar experiences can alleviate feelings of isolation. Open communication with loved ones about feelings and challenges can also foster a supportive environment, helping patients navigate the emotional complexities of living with cirrhosis.

Ultimately, living well with cirrhosis is about taking proactive steps toward health management and lifestyle choices. By prioritizing medical care, nutrition, physical activity, and emotional support, individuals can significantly improve their quality of life. It is essential to remain informed and engaged in one's care while building a supportive network of healthcare providers, family, and friends. With commitment and resilience, patients can manage their condition effectively and continue to lead fulfilling lives despite the challenges posed by cirrhosis.

Author Notes & Acknowledgments

First and foremost, I would like to express my deepest gratitude to the people who inspired and supported me throughout the journey of writing this book. This project would not have been possible without their unwavering belief in me and their invaluable contributions.

To my wife, thank you for your constant encouragement and understanding. Your love and support have been my anchor during the challenging times of researching and writing this book. Your belief in my ability to make a difference in people's lives has been my driving force.

I would also like to disclose that this book contains some renewed artificial intelligence-generated content. I really appreciate very recent technological innovation by outstanding scientists and of course our reader's understanding.

Lastly, I want to express my deepest gratitude to the readers of this book. I sincerely hope the strategies and methods outlined within these pages will provide you with the knowledge and tools needed to truly make your life much better. Your commitment to seeking any good solutions and willingness to explore multiple methods is commendable.

Author Bio

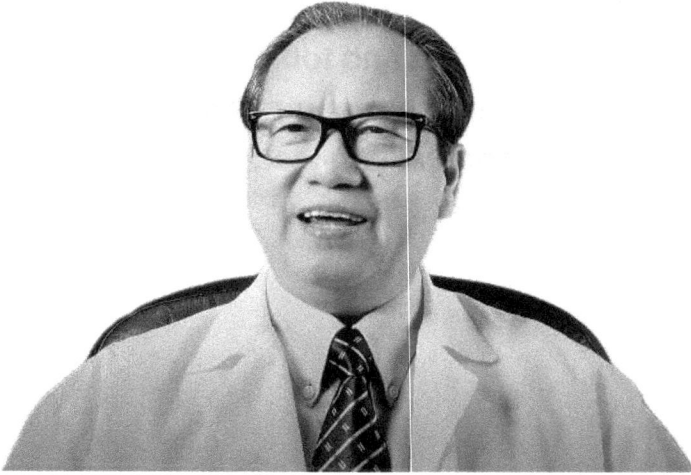

Johnson Wu earned his MD in 1982. With over 40 years of clinical experience, he has worked in hospitals in Zhejiang and Shanghai, China, as well as the Royal Marsden Hospital (part of Imperial College) in London, UK. Upon the recommendation of Sir Aaron Klug, the president of The Royal Society and a Nobel Prize winner in Chemistry, Dr. Wu was honorably awarded a British Royal Society Fellowship. He has published over 100 medical books in many countries and currently practices medicine in Canada.

www.ingramcontent.com/pod-product-compliance
Lightning Source LLC
Chambersburg PA
CBHW060240030426
42335CB00014B/1543